Eye know how

To our parents

Eye know how

Scott Fraser

Friends of Moorfields Research Fellow, Moorfields Eye Hospital, London

Riaz Asaria

Specialist Registrar in Ophthalmology, Moorfields Eye Hospital, London

Chee Kon

Consultant Ophthalmologist, Worthing Hospital, Worthing, West Sussex

BMJ
Books

First published in 2001
by BMJ Books, BMA House, Tavistock Square,
London WC1H 9JR

www.bmjbooks.com

British Library Cataloguing in Publication Data

A catalogue record for this book is available from the British Library

ISBN 0–7279–1413–8

Cover design by Egelnick and Webb, London
Typeset by Academic + Technical Typesetting, Bristol
Printed and bound in Great Britain by J. W. Arrowsmith Ltd, Bristol

Contents

Contents

Preface

Although ophthalmology retains a toe-hold in the undergraduate curriculum, the knowledge gained does not tend to retain a hold in the memory of the postgraduate. This book was written with the intention of giving a helping hand to those whose grip is slipping.

The problem for the non-specialist is that not only does ophthalmology appear to have a wide range of impenetrable conditions, but being able to see these conditions takes a level of skill (i.e. practice) that only examining a large number of eye patients gives. The approach of many ophthalmology books is to use colour pictures to aid in pattern recognition. Whilst this approach can be very useful, these books tend to be large, expensive, and often can only illustrate conditions in their more severe forms. In an attempt to avoid this, our book relies more on using symptoms and simple examination techniques to allow you to make, if not always a diagnosis, a quick assessment of the severity of the condition and of the need for referral.

This book aims to do two things — to show that you do not need fancy equipment to make even some of the more subtle diagnoses and once you have diagnosed them to try to tell you exactly what to do with them. We have tried to cover the common situations that eye conditions present in such as general practice surgeries, accident and emergency departments, minor injury units, optometrists' practices, and the hospital ward.

There are two ways to use this book. Firstly, you can use it as an introduction or refresher for ophthalmology — the first two sections are designed to guide you through the history and examination of eye diseases and although they can be dipped into, are best read in their entirety. Medical, nursing or optometry students may find these useful as an introduction to ophthalmology.

Secondly, the "What you should do" topics are designed for quick access when the patient with that problem is sitting in front of you. The topics purposely concentrate on the common diagnoses and procedures that other ophthalmic books have a tendency to assume knowledge of. Thus it is no accident that there is a large amount of detail regarding corneal foreign body and abrasion but much less on age-related macular degeneration (ARMD) or cataract. Non-ophthalmologists have to definitively deal with foreign bodies or abrasions whereas they do not have to deal with ARMD or cataract, just be able to recognise and refer them.

Hand in hand with this we have tried to make the book readily accessible and there is therefore a detailed contents page, a quick reference guide to common ophthalmic symptoms and one for techniques and procedures. The index is as exhaustive as possible in an attempt to allow speedy access to signs, symptoms, diseases, managements, and treatments. At the end of the book is a glossary of abbreviations and common terms used in ophthalmology — there is a tendency for ophthalmology to disappear into its own hieroglyphics and the glossary is an attempt to decode this.

The essence of the book is that it is a practical guide to ophthalmology. It assumes that the reader has some theoretical knowledge of ophthalmology but no practical experience. The concept we have tried to keep in mind has been to think of ourselves standing behind your shoulder as you deal with the patient with an eye condition at midnight on a Sunday. Further to this concept, we hope to make this book a dynamic creation and if you feel that there are areas that are not covered adequately (or not covered at all) please let us know via the e-mail address: *eyeknowhowonline@hotmail.com.*

N.B. Main referral priorities indicated in the text:
Immediate referral Means the opthalmologist should be
    contacted by telephone so that the patient can be seen
    immediately
Same-day referral Seen within 24 hours
Routine referral Means sending a letter to outpatients

Acknowledgments

We are extremely grateful to the people listed below who very kindly took the time and the trouble to read and review this book. Their suggestions have proved invaluable. Many thanks to Tanveer Asaria, Mike Baines, Glen Brice, Dave Clark, Norman Dudley, James Holt, Pimpra Kon, Helen McClelland, Luke Membrey, Peter Shah, Dilani Siriwardena, Patti Daly and Carey Tierney.

We would also like to thank Mary Banks of BMJ Books for her kindness, encouragement and most of all, her patience.

Finally, we have to thank our wives, Helen, Ismat and Pimpra, for all their support and understanding.

Quick reference — common ophthalmic symptoms

Quick reference — ophthalmic techniques and procedures

Section 1
What you should ask

The ophthalmic history is thought by some to be a contradiction in terms. Ophthalmology is a specialty in which there are a bewildering number of diagnoses — many of which are made through pattern recognition using specialised equipment and thereby appearing to make history taking redundant.

While admittedly there are a few ophthalmologists who have dispensed with history taking altogether, it remains a skill which can pay rich dividends to all practitioners. It is because ophthalmology appears to be available only to those who have mastered its instruments that good history taking is so important to the non-ophthalmologist. This section attempts to show how many diagnoses can be made with the history alone, highlights trigger symptoms that require immediate referral, and tries to deal with the common situations that arise in everyday practice.

The first part of this section puts the ophthalmic consultation within the framework of the classical history, while the second part attempts to show the process of "dynamic" history taking triggered by the patient's symptoms. This section ends by listing the "trigger symptoms" that may be indicative of a specific course of action.

N.B. Main referral priorities indicated in the text:
Immediate referral Means the opthalmologist should be contacted by telephone so that the patient can be seen immediately.
Same-day referral Seen within 24 hours
Routine referral Means sending a letter to outpatients

The structured ophthalmic history

Like medical students approaching their first patient, for those who are unfamiliar with ophthalmology it may be worth using a structured format to begin with. As you gain more confidence, irrelevant areas can be avoided.

The presenting complaint

Like any good history it is important to elicit from the patient the reason why he/she has consulted you, i.e. the presenting complaint. Like any specialty, asking a question such as "What brought you here?" may often receive the response "the ambulance". Conversely, asking the patient "what is wrong with your eyes?" allows the possibility of missing important symptoms.

One needs to devise a way of opening the consultation without making assumptions or inhibiting the patient from actually telling you what symptoms brought him/her to see you. Phrases like "how can I help you?" or "what is worrying you?" put the patient at ease and make him/her more likely to actually answer the question. Of course like other specialties, patients can have multiple symptoms or can spend a lot of time actually getting to the matter they have consulted you about. Again, this is handled like any other consultation — he/she is gently persuaded to prioritise his/her symptoms or to cut short any unnecessary lead up to the problem.

Ophthalmology does have a number of symptoms specific to itself, some of which require prompt action and/or referral. These will be dealt with in the second part of this section when some common presenting symptoms and the subsequent questions that need to be asked regarding these are looked at.

History of the presenting complaint

Again this is as vital as in any other discipline. If a patient complains of a decrease in vision, then it is important to know if this decrease has occurred over a period of months/years when one may think of a cataract requiring routine referral. However, if the decrease has been over say the previous 24 hours then the referral should be made on the same day.

Associated symptoms that started with the presenting complaint are vital. For example, if the sudden decrease in vision was associated with a tender scalp and headache the diagnosis of temporal arteritis would need to be seriously considered.

As in the presenting complaint, gently forcing the patient to be specific about his/her symptoms in terms of time-course, severity, character of pain or visual loss is vital in order to make the diagnosis and to decide on the necessity and speed of referral.

Past ophthalmic history

This is part of the history that non-ophthalmologists will be unfamiliar with, but is often a good indicator of the diagnosis. For example, any patient with a history of uveitis who has a red eye is very likely to be having a recurrence.

Past medical history

As well as taking a past ophthalmic history, a good knowledge of the patient's past medical history may give vital information. For example, in a patient with headache and a history of polmyalgia rheumatica, it would be prudent to think of temporal arteritis. Similarly, a patient who has recently been started on anticholinergic medication and now has ocular pain with reduced vision needs to have acute closed angle glaucoma excluded.

Drug history

It is extremely important to know what drugs the patient is taking — whether systemic, topical or inhaled. There is a huge range of drugs that can have an impact on eye disease and medications for eye disease can have profound systemic effects. Products bought over the counter and those prescribed by alternative practitioners should not be forgotten and often need to be specifically asked about.

General allergies and a history of allergy to any previous eye medications must also be noted.

Systems review

Perhaps not quite as relevant as other parts of the history, as the "pick-up" rate is much less than with a general medical patient. Nonetheless, ophthalmology attracts its mystery diagnoses like any other specialty and in these circumstances a systems review may glean useful information.

Systems review is also important when a patient has an eye disease that can be associated with a systemic disease, e.g. uveitis or scleritis.

Family history

Many ophthalmic diagnoses can be unearthed from the family history (FH). In particular a number of retinal diseases such as retinitis pigmentosa run in families. Similarly, many common diseases such as cataract, glaucoma and squint can run in families. The likely severity of some of these diseases can also be gauged from the FH and it is worth asking if an affected relative became blind or was substantially affected by their visual loss. This will not only give you some indication of the prognosis of your patient, but might be a valuable insight into any worries or fears the patient may have.

The question of consanguinity is also important, as many autosomal recessive conditions have serious eye anomalies as a feature.

Social history

The social history is as important in ophthalmology as in any other branch of medicine. The social circumstances of a patient who may be or may become visually impaired are important in deciding appropriateness of treatment. The patient's ability to instill topical eye preparations and the need for social work input or blind/partial sight registration are essential points to note.

A patient's occupation and hobbies indicate their visual demands (including driving) and may dictate cataract surgery even at a relatively good level of vision.

The dynamic ophthalmic history

The text above outlines the ophthalmic history in terms of classical history structure but this structure is normally abandoned for a more focused, symptom-led history. In reality, eye patients tend to present with a limited number of symptoms (despite the huge range of potential diagnoses), and the following deals with some of the more common symptoms. Management of the various conditions is presented in Section 3.

Presenting complaint: "My eye is red..."

Figure 1.1 indicates some of the symptoms to elicit in the history and the possible diagnoses they represent.

1 **One or both eyes.** Bilateral sticky red eyes — the patient often complains that their eyes are "glued" shut in the mornings — indicates infectious conjunctivitis and this may be viral, bacterial or chlamydial. When these symptoms are unilateral, infectious conjunctivitis is still the most likely diagnosis; however, the index of suspicion should rise for chlamydial conjunctivitis, especially in at-risk groups (i.e. sexually active, genitourinary symptoms).

2 **Itch.** Infectious conjunctivitis causes a gritty sensation, so if itch is the predominant symptom then think of allergic conjunctivitis. In atopic individuals the diagnosis is usually obvious, while those on topical medications may have contact hypersensitivity. Patients with allergic conjunctivitis can have discharge but this tends to be much less than in the infective cases.

3 **Pain.** When the patient complains of pain (rather than dis-comfort/irritation) then alarm bells should ring as a number of potentially serious diagnoses are possible. If the vision is reduced then the patient needs same-day referral. Photophobia can suggest acute anterior uveitis or corneal diseases such as herpes simplex.

4 **Contact lens wearers** with a unilateral red eye need immediate referral to exclude microbial corneal infections.

5 **Chronically, red gritty eyes** tends to suggest blepharitis.

6 **Sudden onset** of a red eye without any other symptoms suggests a subconjunctival haemorrhage. This can be quite dramatic and the patient often needs reassurance. All patients with subcon-junctival haemorrhage need their blood pressure measured.

Presenting complaint: "There's something wrong with my vision..."

Figure 1.2 is a guide to assessing a patient who complains of a reduction in vision. Obviously examination is a vital component of this and how to approach this is detailed in Section 2.

The first question to ask a patient who complains of a decrease in vision is the time-course. **Sudden loss of vision** needs careful

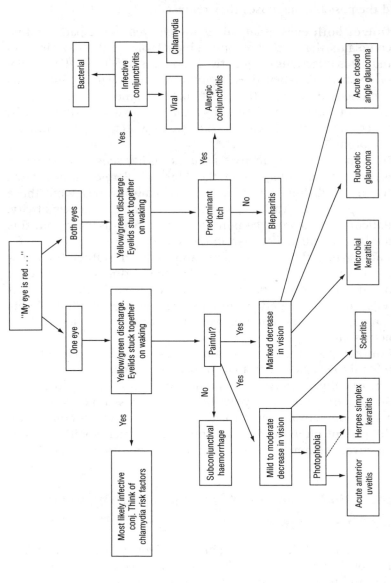

Figure 1.1 Flow diagram for assessing the presenting complaint "My eye is red . . .".

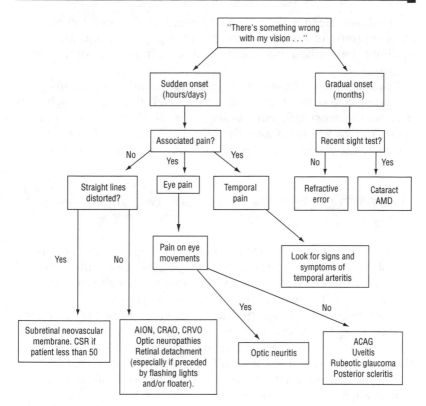

Figure 1.2 Flow diagram for assessing the presenting complaint "There's something wrong with my vision . . .".

definition of how quickly it came on and how long ago it occurred. It is useful to ask the patient when he or she first noticed the decline in vision, as the visual loss (unilateral) may have been present for some time but only noticed when the other eye was shut.

The time-course of the visual loss is extremely important (although should of course be taken in context of other symptoms). A true sudden loss of vision needs immediate referral as it indicates important underlying pathology.

Distortion of straight lines, e.g. door or window frames, is strongly indicative of serious macular pathology and requires same-day referral.

Pain associated with sudden decrease in vision has a number of causes. If the patient feels the pain is coming from the eye itself then closed angle glaucoma, uveitis or scleritis may be diagnostic possibilities. Head and/or temporal pain needs careful evaluation for symptoms of temporal arteritis (see page 17) and an ESR if in doubt. Pain when moving the eye is an important sign of optic neuritis.

Gradual visual decline occurring over months or perhaps years is obviously less likely to need urgent referral. In fact a sight test may be the most efficient management so that simple refractive errors can be excluded and the optometrist can look for signs of cataract, age-related macular degeneration or chronic glaucoma.

Presenting complaint: "*I can see two of everything*..."

Double vision is an important symptom that in itself can be a major disablement to the patient as well as possibly being the herald of important underlying pathology. For this reason all patients with true double vision need early referral to an eye unit.

Many primary care practitioners consider double vision to be a confusing and complex topic consisting of moving pens or pins to different locations and asking the patient questions that the practitioner cannot remember the significance of and cannot remember at the end of the examination anyway. It is, however, far more important to elicit that the patient has true double vision rather than to try to ascertain the cause or which extraocular muscle is affected.

Patients do not, unfortunately, always present with a complaint of "seeing two objects" but, if this symptom is elicited, referral is mandatory.

Children who present with squints tend not to complain of double vision as they quickly suppress one of the images. If they do complain of double vision it is wise to discuss them with an ophthalmologist or community orthoptist on the same day.

A history-taking algorithm is shown in Figure 1.3, but there are three common situations in which double vision occurs:

1 **Related to trauma.** The cause may of course be obvious such as orbital trauma causing a blow-out fracture of the orbital floor or a head injury causing a disruption of control of central eye movements.

It is not unreasonable to refer a patient with a suspected blow-out fracture to a maxillofacial unit — although it is often useful to get an ophthalmic opinion first to check for associated ocular

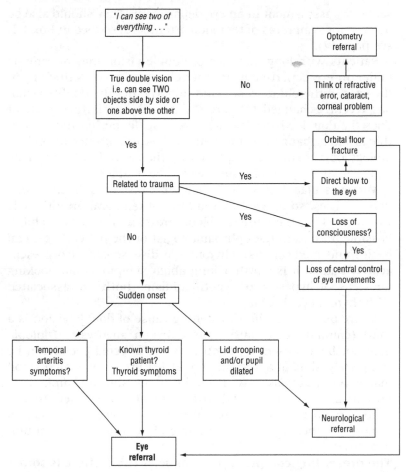

Figure 1.3 Flow diagram for assessing the presenting complaint "I can see two of everything...".

injuries. Double vision following head injury is usually associated with loss of consciousness after the blow and the patient should be treated for their head injury. The diplopia is probably due to disruption of the higher centres of eye movement control and referral to an ophthalmologist is not particularly useful in the acute stages.

2 **The patient who complains of suddenly seeing two of everything.** It is important to ascertain if this is a new symptom or not. Patients with apparently sudden onset of double vision need

same-day assessment in an eye department. They should also be quizzed for symptoms of temporal arteritis (described in Box 1.1, see page 17).

Patients with long histories of double vision may already be under an eye department or other clinics, e.g. endocrinology in the case of thyroid disease. Find out whether the double vision has recently changed (i.e. are the two objects farther apart or does the double vision last for longer spells during the day). If things have changed or the patient is worried, refer to opthal-mology outpatients but explain why the referral is being made and that an early appointment would be justified.

Microvascular disease is a common cause of isolated cranial nerve palsies, so as well as thinking of temporal arteritis it is worth checking the patient's blood pressure. It is also useful, if possible, to inform the ophthalmologist of the patient's general health and medications. Thyroid eye disease can also present acutely and so it is worth asking about symptoms and looking for signs of hyper- and hypothyroidism (**both** are associated with thyroid eye disease).

A rare but acutely life-threatening cause of double vision is a third (cranial) nerve palsy caused by an aneurysm. Diplopia may not be a presenting feature as the affected eyelid can be completely shut and the additional feature of a dilated pupil makes the diagnosis easy. If the lid is not shut but diplopia is present and the pupil is dilated (both of acute onset) then a third nerve palsy needs to be ruled out — whether it is painful or not. In either case immediate referral to a neurosurgical unit is necessary.

3 **The presenting complaint is a vague "I think there is some-thing wrong with my vision".** This can of course be difficult and may indicate a number of different symptoms. This is discussed on page 20. Sometimes it is necessary to go through a full formal history as described at the beginning of this chapter in order to gain an insight into the true nature of the symptoms.

If double vision appears to be the presenting symptom, once again try to ascertain from the patient whether he/she is actually seeing two objects — either side by side or one on top of another. It may help if the patient draws what he/she can see. Patients who are seeing an "edge" on objects caused by uncorrected refractive errors or cataracts can confuse this with double vision — this does not need same-day referral and the patient can safely be sent to an optometrist.

Finally, remember that anyone with double vision should be told not to drive and it is important to warn the patient to inform the DVLA.

Presenting complaint: "*Something hit me in the eye...*"

As with any trauma anywhere on the body it is **imperative** that a full and accurate history is taken. It is too easy to avoid getting the patient to specify the exact nature of the eye injury they sustained and sometimes the patient may be deliberately avoiding the truth.

Trauma history matters because it tells you what forces were acting on the eye and in what places, allowing you to gauge the probable extent of the damage and its site. Once you have defined the nature of the injury you need to ask about associated symptoms:

1 Has your vision gone down?
2 Are you seeing two of things?
3 Is your eye uncomfortable or light sensitive?

A deterioration in vision needs ophthalmic referral to check for perforating injuries, hyphaema, retinal damage or detachment or optic nerve trauma. Double vision after trauma is dealt with above.

A painful or photophobic eye after trauma can indicate a variety of problems, from simple corneal abrasions to major ocular trauma or secondary raised intraocular pressure (IOP). If the associated trauma has been significant, same day ophthalmic referral is advisable.

It needs to be stressed, as above, that it is important to define the degree of trauma. Common examples of ocular trauma and their likely sequelae are discussed below; it is of course necessary to assess these in the context of other symptoms and examination findings:

1 **Wind-blown foreign bodies** (FBs) are unlikely to cause serious injury. They also have a propensity to appear under the upper lid.
2 An ocular FB sustained when hitting **metal onto metal**, e.g. hammer and chisel or drilling metal, gives the highest incidence

of intraocular penetration because of the high velocity and small, sharp fragments. All metal on metal injuries need AP and lateral orbital X-rays, although this can lead to false positives and negatives.

3 The three rules of treatment of **ocular burns** (acid, alkaline or thermal) are: first — irrigate, second — irrigate and third — irrigate. This means anyone who gives a history — however vague — of chemical or thermal injury needs irrigation of the affected eye (this is described on p. 135).

4 Ocular injuries caused by **glass**, unless very minor, need to be X-rayed (the amount of lead in the glass determines how radiolucent the glass is) and same day referral to an eye department, as it is relatively easy for the inexperienced examiner to miss intraocular glass.

Presenting complaint: *"My eyelids are swollen..."*

Swollen eyelids range from the very minor to the life threatening and need careful evaluation. The main differential is between allergy and infection. Allergic lid swelling (unless part of a systemic anaphylaxis) is annoying but not serious to the patient. With lid infection, however, the possibility of orbital cellulitis and subsequent cavernous sinus thrombosis needs to be kept in mind.

The symptoms that help differentiate allergic and infective lid swelling are listed in Table 1.1. A red **tender** lid must be assumed to be infected and treated appropriately in an attempt to reduce

Table 1.1 Symptoms that help differentiate allergic and infective lid swelling

Allergic symptoms	Infective symptoms
Itch	Pain
Bilateral	Unilateral
Associated with other atopy/allergies	Tender to touch
Very sudden onset	Yellow–green discharge
Systemically well	May be systemically unwell
Vision unaffected	Vision decreased
May be a slight stringy discharge	May be a history of sinus disease
	Diplopia
	History of lacrimal disease/watering eye
	Redness

the potential for spread. In children and the elderly, hospital admission may be necessary.

A number of typical presentations of lid disease, which can point to specific diagnoses, are grouped under the headings allergic and infective.

Allergic

1 **Acute lid and conjunctival swelling.** This occurs very suddenly after exposure to a large concentration of antigen, e.g. walking across a field. It usually occurs in spring or summer, is often bilateral and is characterised by its speed of onset which is usually over a number of minutes. The lids and conjunctiva become very swollen — the latter can protrude from between the lids and is described by witnesses as "a jelly coming out of the eye". This condition is one which causes great panic to all concerned, but because it is often settled by the time the patient is seen it is best recognised by its symptoms. No treatment is required except reassurance.
2 **Atopic** individuals often have lid swelling that comes and goes with their other manifestations. Lid swelling is usually bilateral, chronic and itch is the major symptom. Predominantly unilateral disease can be confusing but again itch is the symptom that is most useful in making the diagnosis.
3 Perhaps one of the commonest causes of a unilateral swollen lid is **an allergy to eye medications.** It is always therefore worth asking these patients if they are taking any prescribed or over the counter medications in their eyes. Treatment involves stopping the medication or changing the preparation; however, if this has been prescribed by an ophthalmologist it is wise to consult the department first.

Infective

1 Small localised lid swellings are usually due to blocked meibomian glands (**chalazia**) and treatment is with hot bathing and the majority settle spontaneously. If there is any suspicion of surrounding cellulitis, systemic antibiotics are indicated — eye drops or ointments are ineffective.
2 Lacrimal sac infections (**dacrocystitis**) with surrounding redness can appear as lid swelling but need aggressive antibiotic treatment.

3 **Preseptal cellulitis**. This is swelling of upper and lower lids that
  is all in front of the orbital septum, i.e. is anatomically isolated
  and does not have access to the posterior orbit, cavernous
  sinus and brain. Because the infection is limited the patients
  affected are systemically well, vision is normal, there is no diplopia (double vision) and the pain is mild. It is not life threatening
  but should be treated aggressively (see page 93) to prevent the
  infection breaking through the septum.
4 **Orbital cellulitis**. When infection spreads behind the septum the
  patient is often systemically upset, vision declines as the optic
  nerve is affected and there may be diplopia as extraocular
  muscles are affected or from the proptosis (abnormal protrusion
  of the eye). This is a medical emergency (see page 93).

Presenting complaint: *"I've got a headache, but I think it's my eye . . ."*

The purpose of the history in the context of this book is to separate
headache caused by eye disease from headache of non-ocular
origin. The number of patients who localise their head pain to the
eye, supra-orbital or retro-orbital region is high — although unsur-
prising as they all share a common trigeminal sensory innervation.
However, the proportion of patients who present with headache of
ocular origin without other pointers of eye disease is relatively
small. In other words the patient who complains of headache but
actually has ocular disease is usually easy to spot.

Eye diseases that can present with headache

In theory, any cause of ocular pain can present with headache. In
reality, there are certain ocular pathologies which seem to have a
propensity to present in this way:

- Acute closed angle glaucoma.
- Acute anterior uveitis.
- Scleritis.
- Endophthalmitis.
- Dacrocystitis.
- Temporal arteritis.
- Optic neuritis (retrobulbar neuritis).

Non-ocular disease that can present to the ophthalmologist

The other side of the coin is those diseases that not uncommonly present as eye disease when in fact the pathology is non-ocular in origin:

- Temporal arteritis.
- Sinus disease.
- Migraine.
- Meningeal irritation.
- Tension headache.

An algorithm to aid in the differentiation of these conditions is shown in Figure 1.4. Perhaps the two most useful symptoms to separate ocular and non-ocular origins of head pain are decrease in vision and an injected (i.e. red) eye. If both these features are present it strongly suggests ocular pathology such as **acute closed angle glaucoma (ACAG)**, **acute anterior uveitis (AAU)**, **scleritis** or **endophthalmitis**. It may also be possible to elicit a history of haloes around lights that points to ACAG. Scleritis can present without a red eye (typically posterior scleritis) or with normal vision (typically anterior scleritis), thus it is a diagnosis that can be easy to miss.

Dacrocystitis can present with periorbital pain but often further questioning can pinpoint the pain to the inner canthus. A preceding history of a watering eye (for months or years) and recurrent infections is common and suggestive of dacrocystitis.

Unilateral pain when moving the eye even without other symptoms is suggestive of early **optic neuritis.** If other symptoms such as decreased visual acuity and colour perception abnormalities do not follow within a few days then the diagnosis should be reconsidered. In patients with symptoms of active sinus disease (see below) consider CT scanning immediately to rule out the possibility of sphenoidal sinusitis causing the symptoms (a rare but potentially curable cause).

In any patient with headache, who is over 50 years of age, **temporal arteritis** must be excluded. The most specific way to do this is via the symptoms — these are described in Box 1.1. Although an ESR is a very useful confirmatory test it has a high rate of false positives and negatives.

Sinus disease can often present with pain in and around the eye (which is not surprising given the close proximity of the sinuses to the orbit) and can be difficult to diagnose. A past history of sinus

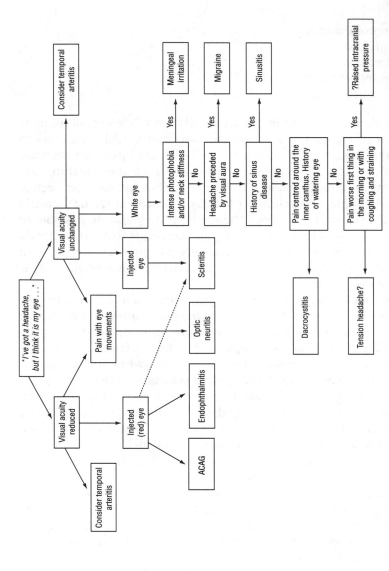

Figure 1.4 Flow diagram for assessing the presenting complaint "I've got a headache but I think it's my eye….". (See text for abbreviations.)

Box 1.1 Symptoms of temporal arteritis

This is a disease that strikes fear into all ophthalmologists as the sufferer can lose vision in both eyes very quickly. Most practitioners tend to recognise the classic symptoms of TA shown below:

- Unilateral headache.
- Very tender temple.
- Pain when brushing hair.

However there are other symptoms, perhaps not so well recognised, that may point to the diagnosis:

- Pain when eating (involvement of lingual artery) sometimes called "jaw claudication".
- Night sweats ("my night clothes are soaked when I wake in the mornings").
- Malaise.
- Poor appetite.

It is also helpful to remember that temporal arteritis almost never occurs in patients under the age of 50 years.

---

disease helps (along with the question "have you had a pain like this before?"), pain maximal over the sinus, nasal discharge and a recent upper respiratory tract infection (URTI) push the diagnosis towards sinusitis. Sinus infection can spread into the orbit and cause an orbital cellulitis — signs include systemic upset, decreased vision and proptosis.

It is not uncommon for patients with **migraine** to present with the ocular symptoms like visual aura or transient hemianopia. The clues to the diagnosis are often given by the presence of an aura, a headache that begins only after the other symptoms have gone, and a past or family history of migraine. Any patient who has an apparent first migraine over the age of 50 or who has symptoms that do not pass should be referred to a neurologist.

Patients with **meningeal irritation** (e.g. meningitis, encephalitis, subarachnoid haemorrhage) are usually obvious but in the early stages of the disease, headache and photophobia can predominate and the patient referred for ophthalmic assessment. Clues to the real diagnosis may be subtle, such as slight behavioural changes, slight systemic upset or mild neck stiffness. If the changes are subtle the patient may be reviewed later or relatives given very precise instructions on what further symptoms to look for and to bring the patient back immediately.

Periocular pain with no other symptoms may be put down to **tension headache** especially if it occurs towards the end of the day or after heavy book work and there are no other suspicious symptoms. However, note that early presbyopia and/or convergence problems can give the same symptoms, so it may be worth suggesting these patients see their optometrist.

Presenting complaint: *"There's nothing wrong with my eyes but my optometrist sent me..."*

One of the commonest referral routes for patients is a routine sight test. The patient may have visited the optometrist because of specific symptoms and the optometrist's input is often very helpful. Many optometrists now use their skills for more than just refraction (testing for glasses), inevitably meaning that symptomless ophthalmic disease is likely to be picked up and referred to the primary care practitioner. This means that some patients will bring a GOS18 form* with them and want to know what is wrong with them and what you are going to do about it? A question you may in fact be asking yourself.

For the time being, the system of ophthalmic referral in the UK means that if an optometrist diagnoses any eye disease or abnormality in a patient he/she is bound to refer the patient to their GP. This may be for a number of reasons, most of which should be clear on the referral form. It is therefore important for:

1 The referring optometrist to make clear the reason for referral.
2 For the GP or A&E personnel who receive the referral, to read the GOS18 form to see what the optometrist actually wants.

The points under the following four headings illustrate the common reasons for referral from optometrists and may be of some help.

---

* GOS18 is the form on which an optometrist reports a patient's findings to the GP. The GP then refers the patient to an ophthalmologist by onward referral of this form. There is also a space on this form for the GP to add his/her comments or findings.

Significant eye disease picked up

When this occurs the optometrist states the presumptive diagnosis and suggests referral to the hospital eye service (HES). In the asymptomatic patient this is usually for POAG (primary open angle glaucoma) or early AMD (age-related macular degeneration); both these need referral, the former for possible treatment and follow-up, the latter for explanation and advice. By definition, it is not necessary to refer all symptomless cataracts — it is worth talking to the patient and to see if they want referral. Some patients are adamant they do not want an operation and therefore it is necessary to discuss this with the patient prior to referral to avoid wasting the patient's and ophthalmologist's time.

A patient in whom referral to the HES is made on an optometrist's recommendations may still gain from being referred via the GP as it allows the ophthalmologist to have a clearer picture of the patient's general health and social history. For this reason it is always worth filling in the part of the GOS18 form that is available for this purpose.

Informing the GP of findings

Some optometrists let the GP know of anything abnormal they find in the patient but do not recommend referral. This can put the GP in a difficult position as he/she often has less eye knowledge than the referring optometrist. Examples of this may be such things as a few drusen at the macula, a single cotton-wool spot or early lens opacities.

Most of these things are difficult to find discussed in textbooks, as they are not conditions in themselves and are generally of no significance. Unless you are confident about the findings the best thing to do is to contact the referring optometrist and ask for further details or to ring up an eye department or casualty who are usually pleased to deal with the query by telephone.

Once you have a better idea of the condition and what to do with it, it may be a good idea to contact the patient to ensure the findings are understood.

Asking for systemic evaluation

A small number of referrals will be requests from optometrists for certain examinations or investigations based on their findings.

For example there may be a request for blood pressure measurement in a patient with silver-wiring of retinal arterioles or recurrent subconjunctival haemorrhages, or a blood sugar in a young patient with early lens opacities.

Usually these patients do not need referral but the findings can be discussed with the optometrist or an ophthalmologist.

Optometrist unsure about the findings

The optometrist may have found an abnormality but be unsure of its significance. This often requires starting from scratch with a full history and examination and further discussion with an ophthalmologist.

Presenting complaint: *"I'm not sure what it is but my eyes don't seem right..."*

Whatever the body system involved most practitioners will experience the famous heart-sink when the patient's presenting comment is "...but it doesn't feel right". Consultations such as this have a tendency to be overlong and to leave patient and practitioner unsatisfied. An approach to taking the history in these patients is provided here, it attempts to pinpoint if the problem is eye related and how serious it is.

It may be useful to use a series of steps in the history in an attempt to refine the patient's true symptoms:

Step 1: Is it really an eye problem that the patient has?

Step 2: If you are satisfied that the patient's symptoms are ocular, what category do they fall into? The main categories are those mentioned in this section already, e.g. is your eye irritable/uncomfortable? Do you have double vision or has your vision gone down? It is of course vitally important not to shoe-horn patients into incorrect diagnoses just to make life simpler. This leads to inappropriate treatment and to missed diagnoses.

Step 3: If the patient's symptoms remain difficult to pin down then it may be necessary to use the structured history described earlier in this chapter. This is general enough to pick up the majority of eye problems, but also has the advantage of eliciting symptoms that may not be ocular but which may give clues to the underlying problem.

Step 4: Although it was stated at the start of this section that most ophthalmic diagnoses could be made by taking a good history, there are certain patients in which it cannot and the examination makes the diagnoses. This often occurs in those patients whose symptoms do not fit into a diagnostic category and a careful examination is essential. These patients are often aware something is wrong but are unable to articulate what it is, e.g. visual field loss, subtle ocular motility problems or a subtle decrease in vision.

Simple rules to make life easier

This section lists some important symptoms that should trigger certain actions — usually referral. Although the symptoms do not guarantee the associated diagnosis, they are specific enough for those without specialist knowledge or equipment to refer to an eye department. (**Note:** Immediate referral means contacting the eye department and arranging for the patient to attend immediately. Same-day referral means that the patient should usually be seen within 24 hours.)

- **Uveitis** patients who feel they are starting an attack should be referred (the same day) whatever the signs.
- Any patient who reports a change in **floaters** (i.e. new onset or recent increase) needs same-day referral.
- Patients who complain of recent onset of **haloes/rainbows** around lights need immediate referral to rule out narrow angle glaucoma.
- Patients who complain of **distortion of straight lines** (e.g. door frames or window frames) need urgent, same-day ophthalmic referral to rule out a neovascular membrane at the macula.
- Any patient who has **recently undergone intraocular surgery** of any type and complains of increasing redness or reduction in vision needs immediate referral to exclude endophthalmitis.
- Patients who have had a **trabeculectomy** can remain at risk of infection long after the operation and require referral with the above symptoms.
- Sudden onset of **double vision** requires immediate referral to an ophthalmologist.

- Any suggestion of a **chemical injury** needs irrigation before a full history or examination is taken.
- **Contact lens wearers** with a unilateral red, painful eye need same-day referral to an eye casualty department.
- Painful or tender **lid swelling** should be presumed to be infective in origin.
- **Pain with eye movements** is indicative of optic neuritis.
- **Photophobia** is almost always a significant symptom. If it is bilateral think of meningitis, if it is unilateral think of keratitis or uveitis.
- **Sudden loss of vision** is never refractive in origin.
- **"Getting older"** is not a cause of decreasing vision, there must be a reason for it — correctable or not.
- Patients who have previously **lost vision in one eye** almost always should be referred for an ophthalmic opinion if they experience anything but the most trivial symptoms in their remaining eye.
- No **child** with an eye problem should leave the consultation without a diagnosis.
- Those who have **had injuries involving glass** should be assumed to have a perforating injury until proven otherwise.
- Any patient with **sudden or intermittent loss of vision** needs to be questioned for symptoms of temporal arteritis (listed in Box 1.1).

Section 2
What you should see

It is possible to diagnose many eye diseases quickly and accurately **without** specialist skill and equipment. For the non-specialist, rather than making a definitive diagnosis it is more important to be able to elicit the signs that indicate when to refer a case for specialist management. Of course, as in any branch of medicine, examination findings are only relevant in the context of the history.

As in the previous section, those inexperienced in ophthalmology may well prefer a structured stepwise approach to the examination and as more experience is gained to direct the examination more towards those parts of the eye that may have produced the patient's symptoms.

The important components to the examination for a complete eye examination and the order in which they can be tested are:

1 Visual acuity.
2 Colour vision.
3 Visual field testing.
4 Ocular movements.
5 Pupil reactions.
6 Examination of the external eye.
7 Optic disc and retina.

N.B. Main referral priorities indicated in the text:
Immediate referral Means the opthalmologist should be contacted by telephone so that the patient can be seen immediately
Same-day referral Seen within 24 hours
Routine referral Means sending a letter to outpatients

Visual acuity

No ophthalmic examination is valid without measuring the distance visual acuity of each eye separately. Near vision is less often measured but can be just as useful.

Visual acuity can be affected by:

1 Refractive errors — myopia ("short-sightedness"), hypermetropia ("long-sightedness") or astigmatism.
2 Any obstruction to light passage through the visual axis (e.g. cataract or corneal scarring).
3 Abnormalities of the retina (e.g. macular degeneration or retinal detachment).
4 Abnormalities of the optic nerve (e.g. optic neuritis or anterior ischaemic optic neuropathy, temporal arteritis and cortical blindness).
5 Abnormalities of the higher visual centres (e.g. a pituitary tumour pressing on the optic chiasm or occipital lobe infarct).

A normal visual acuity can exclude a number of, but not all, serious eye diseases.

The Snellen chart

Visual acuity is usually measured using printed visual test objects called optotypes. The Snellen test chart and its modifications are most commonly used in the clinical setting for measuring distance visual acuity. The commercially available Snellen chart consists of printed black letters of various sizes with an illuminated background.

In the Snellen system, the visual acuity is denoted by a fraction:

1 The **numerator** indicates **the distance separating the patient and the test chart**.
2 The **denominator** indicates the distance at which **eyes with normal visual acuity** should see those letters.
3 Distances are expressed in metres in Europe and feet in the USA.
4 Good vision in the UK would be denoted as 6/6 and the same patient would be 20/20 in the USA.
5 So for example a visual acuity of 6/36 is a poor visual acuity and means that the patient's eye sees a letter at 6 metres when a "normal" eye would be able to see the same letter at 36 metres.

Table 2.1 Approximate equivalents of Snellen visual acuity (VA) and near vision

Distance vision		Near vision
		(Times New Roman at 35 cm)
Snellen VA (m)	Snellen VA (ft)	
6/6	20/20	
6/7.5	20/25	N5
6/10	20/32	N6
6/12	20/40	
6/15	20/50	
6/18	20/64	
6/24	20/80	
6/30	20/100	N7
6/36	20/125	N9
6/48	20/160	
6/60	20/200	N12
6/90	20/300	N14
6/120	20/400	N18
6/240	20/800	N24

6 These visual acuity measurements are usually printed underneath the Snellen letters.

The numerator could in fact be any distance (e.g. 3/9 would indicate that the visual acuity was tested at 3 metres) but, rather than moving the patient to various distances, the standard Snellen test chart employs difference **sizes** of test letters while the patient is placed at a **fixed distance** of 6 metres (20 feet) from the test type (Table 2.1). The standard chart has a series of letters of decreasing size either singly or printed in rows — each row indicating a different visual acuity. From the top row down:

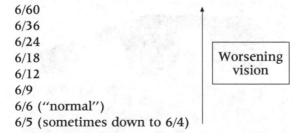

6/60
6/36
6/24
6/18
6/12
6/9
6/6 ("normal")
6/5 (sometimes down to 6/4)

Worsening vision

Modifications of the chart for children and the illiterate (e.g. pictures instead of letters) are also available. Snellen charts can be illuminated from behind (i.e. an opaque chart) or the black letters can be printed on a piece of cardboard with no background illumination (the latter being much cheaper).

How to measure the distance visual acuity

The testing room needs to be well illuminated before commencing the test, i.e. check the visual acuity with the room lights on. Each eye is tested in turn; ask the patient to cover the other eye with the palm of his/her hand over a closed eyelid (beware: make sure the patient is not seeing between the fingers!). The eye can also be covered by a piece of paper or a purpose-made occluder (Figure 2.1). Visual acuity should be measured:

1 Unaided, i.e. without glasses or contact lenses.
2 Aided, i.e. with **distance** glasses — or the distance portion of bifocals (or contact lens if appropriate).
3 With a pinhole. A pinhole is a small opening in an opaque shield through which the patient attempts to read the chart. They are available commercially, usually with an occluder (Figure 2.1), but can be quickly and simply constructed by sticking a pin or pen-tip through a piece of cardboard or paper. Testing the vision using a pinhole can indicate that the patient's reduced vision is due to an uncorrected error of refraction, i.e. the patient requires distance glasses (or if the patient wears them already, they need updating). The advantage of the pinhole

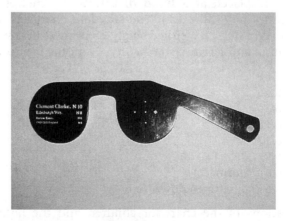

Figure 2.1 A purpose-made occluder.

vision is that any reduction in vision with the pinhole in place is more likely to be pathological than refractive, e.g. cataract, retinal detachment, age-related macular degeneration (ARMD).

When reading the chart, the patient should be instructed to read from the top row (6/60) down to the last row he/she can see. The last correctly read row is then recorded as the best visual acuity. If the patient can only manage to read some of the letters from a particular row (e.g. 6/18 row), this should be recorded as the visual acuity of the previous fully correctly read row (in this case 6/24) plus the number of letters the patient managed to read from the partially read row (e.g. 6/24 + 2). An alternative way of recording this is to note down the visual acuity of the partially read row (6/18) minus the number of letters the patient missed.

If the patient cannot see the top letter (6/60), the visual acuity is worse than 6/60. The patient can be moved closer to the chart and the visual acuity measured as before and the numerator is changed from 6 to that distance, i.e. if they can only see the top letter at 4 metres the visual acuity would be denoted as 4/60. The closest a patient needs to be moved is to 1 metre and the numerator becomes 1/60.

If the patient is unable to see the top letter at 1 metre, then the next step is to hold up a random numbers of fingers at a distance of around 1 metre and ask the patient to indicate how many fingers are being held up. This is done three times and if the patient manages to indicate the number of fingers correctly, the visual acuity is recorded as "count fingers" (CF or CFS).

If the patient is unable to distinguish fingers, hold out the hand (palm facing the patient) about a third of a metre from the patient and move the whole hand. The patient is instructed to indicate to you (e.g. by saying "yes") when he/she can detect this hand move-ment. Move and stop moving your hand at random on three occasions. The vision of the eye is recorded as "hand-movement" (HM or HMS) if the patient accurately indicates this movement.

If the vision is worse than HM, light from a pen-torch is directed to the eye and the patient asked whether they are aware of the light. It is important to make sure that the fellow eye is adequately covered — shutting the eyelid is not enough to exclude light and must be supplemented by the palm of the hand (your hand if pos-sible) over the closed eye. The vision is recorded as "perception of light" (PL) if the patient is able to perceive it, otherwise, the vision is recorded as "no perception of light" (NPL).

It is not common to come across patients with NPL — although colloquially this is used to mean blind, in reality the definition of blindness is more complex (see "Guidelines for blind and partial sight registration", pages 200–202). The word "blind" is best avoided when testing visual acuity as it has various legal and socio-logic definitions.

Near visual acuity

The measurement of near acuity is usually less precise than distance visual acuity and is not usually measured unless for a specific indication requiring it, e.g. when the patient complains of specific problems with reading or a Snellen chart is not available/convenient.

The commonest method used is the commercially available book of printed passages with black letters printed on a white back-ground. The letters are printed in Times Roman typeface with increasing font sizes of 5 pt, 6 pt, 8 pt, 10 pt, 12 pt, 14 pt, 18 pt, 24 pt, 36 pt and 48 pt. (See Table 2.1 for approximate Snellen equivalents.)

The reason that the near visual acuity is less precise than dis-tance visual acuity is because the test conditions tend to be more variable. Try to standardise your near vision testing conditions:

1 Use good lighting conditions, the room lights should be on and if possible an angle-poise lamp should be directed from behind the patient's shoulder making sure it does not cast a shadow or dazzle the patient.
2 The patient should have their normal reading glasses on if they use them or use the lower portion of their bifocals — you are attempting to determine the patient's best reading acuity so the patient can use whatever he/she finds gives the best vision. Remember that some myopes (shortsighted) will take their glasses OFF to improve their reading (see "Optics and refraction for beginners", pages 198–200).
3 Ask the patient to read the print from a distance that he/she finds comfortable. If the reading glasses are appropriate the patient will hold the text at around a third of a metre. If the reading glasses are too weak (or they actually need reading glasses) they will attempt to focus the print by holding the text **farther away**.
4 The near visual acuity is recorded as the smallest type the patient can read. The size of the type is printed above the passages which

the examiner can read off (e.g. size 14 pt is recorded as "N 14", N being the abbreviation for "near").

5 Test with both eyes open and then test one eye at a time.

6 If you don't have access to a near visual acuity test, a passage in a newspaper can be used. Standard newsprint is (not headlines or subheadings) the approximate equivalent of N8 on the standard reading test.

Portable Snellen

An alternative method of measuring near visual acuity, albeit less popular, is the reduced Snellen test. This has the same principle as and is recorded in the same way as the Snellen distance chart except that the letters are reduced to one-seventeenth of the normal size and are meant to be read at a distance of a third of a metre and the patient wears his/her reading glasses if required.

The visual acuity is recorded as for the normal Snellen's acuity. This chart can be useful as it is cheap, pocket-sized and portable, and therefore particularly useful for testing visual acuity at the bedside or the patient's home. It also has the advantage that the acuity is expressed in a way that is generally understood by most practitioners. A reduced Snellen test chart is shown on page 216.

Assessing the patient complaining of visual distortion

An important visual symptom that requires specific testing measures is distortion ("kinks") in the vision.

Ophthalmologists use the Amsler chart to test for visual distortion. This consists of horizontal and vertical straight black lines printed as a grid on a piece of white paper (Figure 2.2). A black spot is printed in the middle of the grid. The patient is instructed to look at the black spot (one eye at a time) from a distance of one-third of a metre and indicate to the practitioner whether any of the grid-lines are distorted (Figure 2.3).

Even without an Amsler chart, there is a simple test that can indicate the presence of visual distortion. Testing each eye in turn, ask the patient to look at a vertical door or window frame and report if there is any disruption, distortion or interruption in the continuity of the line (Figure 2.4). Alternatively, some ophthalmoscopes have

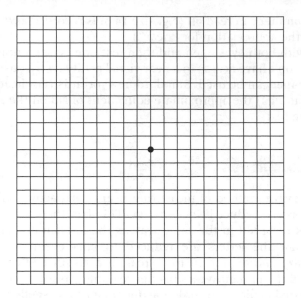

Figure 2.2 The Amsler chart.

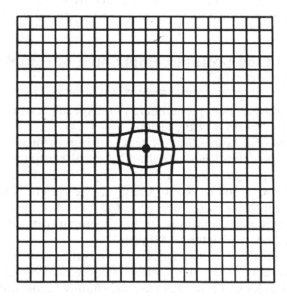

Figure 2.3 A central defect in the Amsler grid, caused by a small lesion in the macular area that has distorted both the horizontal and vertical lines.

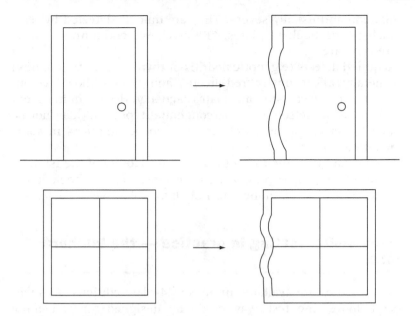

Figure 2.4 The presence of distortion can be elicited by asking the patient (one eye at a time) to look at a straight line and asking them if the line is distorted or parts of it are missing. A door or window frame can be used for this.

a vertical strip as a choice of target. If the ophthalmoscope is used in the normal way and the patient is instructed to look straight into the light they can be asked to describe any distortions or "wiggles" in the line. Distortion is a very important symptom, usually indicating pathology involving the macula and any patient found to have it needs same-day ophthalmic referral.

Colour vision

Colour vision testing and its abnormalities can be complex and full of difficult to remember jargon. Fortunately for the non-ophthalmologist this can be reduced to some basic principles:

1 Colour vision defects can be congenital or acquired.
2 Almost all congenital colour vision defects (all X-linked recessive) are "red-green". This affects approximately 8% of the male population (therefore quite common!) and 0.4% of the female population. Congenital colour vision defects are invariably

bilateral and usually severe. They are quickly detected by tests such as the Ishihara plates. "Blue-yellow" **congenital** defects are very rare.

3 Acquired defects (e.g. optic neuritis or thyroid optic neuropathy) generally affect **both** "red-green" and "blue-yellow" colour vision. However Ishihara plates actually detect quite gross colour vision defects (i.e. the congenital type) and may not be able to detect the mild defects that can be produced in some acquired defects.

4 Having said this, the ease of use and availability of the Ishihara plates (they can be purchased from most medical bookshops) make them the commonest test of all for colour vision defects.

Colour vision testing in practice — the Ishihara plates

Ishihara plates are available in 36- or 24-plate editions. As mentioned above, the test was originally designed for congenital colour vision defects and is a very good test for severe "red-green" defects. It is not a good test for:

1 "Blue-yellow" defects (it does not have "blue-yellow" plates).
2 Acquired colour vision defects in a patient who already has a congenital defect. A patient who has a congenital defect ("red-green") will fail the test and if he/she then develops an acquired defect ("blue-yellow" or "red-green"), the Ishihara plates would not give any further information.
3 Mild colour vision defects.

Unfortunately, it is the only widely available test and therefore has, over the years, been used to test for acquired defects. Be aware that the results from the test are crude but that the test is easy to use and can provide some useful indication of gross "red-green" colour vision defects, especially when one eye is compared with its fellow.

The instructions that come with the Ishihara plates are complicated and usually do not add a great deal to the information obtained if the test is used in the quicker way described below:

1 The test should be conducted in daylight or a brightly lit room (use an angle-poise lamp if necessary). It assumes that the examiner has normal colour vision. The patient should wear

reading glasses if he/she normally does and the plates held at a convenient reading distance for the patient. Each eye is tested in turn.

2 The first plate is shown to the patient. The patient should be told that he/she should see a number (no. 12) and you want him/her to continue to name the number as you flip through the plates one at a time. The first plate is a test plate and all patients (including those with colour vision defects) with reasonable visual acuity (~6/36 or better) will be able to read the number correctly. If the patient is unable to read the first plate, for whatever the reason, the test is abandoned.

3 Continue to show the rest of the plates as soon as the first plate is read correctly, giving the patient about 5 seconds to read each plate. Show only the plates that you can see a number on yourself and skip those on which you cannot see a number. There should be 25 such plates in the 36-plate version. You do not have to show all 25 plates. For example, you could show 10 plates and score the test according to how many plates the patient has read correctly out of 10 plates, e.g. 10/10 or 1/10 (never 0/10 as the test plate must have been seen for the rest of the test to be performed).

4 If you have colour vision defect yourself, you may not be able to read the plates correctly and you will need to refer to the instructions that come with the chart.

Visual field testing

Visual field testing provides extremely important information and is a vital skill to master. Detailed visual field analysis (e.g. for patients with glaucoma) requires sophisticated machinery beyond the scope of this book, but gross visual defects (e.g. most neurological defects) can be detected quickly using the confrontation method.

How to test the visual field

1 Sit facing the patient about 1 metre (roughly arm's length) away. Make sure your head and eyes are at roughly the same height as the patient's. Cover your right eye with your right hand and instruct the patient to cover the eye directly opposite to the one you are covering, i.e. their left eye with the left hand. Alternate this for the other eye. Both you and the patient should use the

palm of the hand rather than the fingers to prevent inadvertently looking through.

2 The patient is instructed to look directly into your uncovered eye (i.e. when the patient's left eye is tested, the patient should be looking at the your right eye).

3 Think of the visual field in four quadrants. There is an anatomical basis to this and it makes both the examination and recording of the findings more logical. The four quadrants are:

Supratemporal	Supranasal
Infratemporal	Infranasal

Note: The results of the visual field examination are drawn on paper as the **patient sees them.** Thus the example shown above must be for the **left eye.** This is convenient as any defects you find on examination, when written down as you find them, automatically represent this.

4 To test the visual field present a random number of fingers from your hand to each of the four quadrants of the patient's visual field shown above. Use only one, two, five or no fingers (clenched fist) and ask the patient to count the number of fingers presented — remember to keep your hand still when presenting the fingers and to make sure that the patient's eye does not move.

5 Hold your fingers roughly halfway between yourself and the patient and remember you are using your own visual field as a control — if you cannot see your fingers then the patient will be unlikely to see them either and you need to bring your hand nearer to the centre. Following the notation system shown above, an example of how a normal result would be **written down:**

	Patient's left eye:			Patient's right eye:		
	CF	CF		CF	CF	
Temporal			Patient's			Temporal
	CF	CF	nose	CF	CF	

CF = count fingers

This method will pick up many of the gross field defects such as homonymous hemianopias.

6 A more sensitive method is to buy a hatpin with a 3- or 5-mm diameter white tip. The white target is introduced diagonally from the periphery of the vision towards the center.

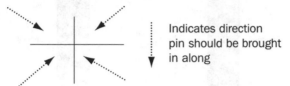

Indicates direction pin should be brought in along

The patient is instructed to indicate (e.g. by saying "yes") as soon as he/she sees the **white target**. The patient is **not** to indicate when he/she sees only the **movement of the your hand**. Record the result using the same notation described above.

7 If the vision is very poor and the patient is unable to make out individual fingers, introduce your moving hand — usually a waving hand diagonally from the periphery (i.e. with your arm extended as far as it can) towards the centre of the vision. Ask the patient to say "yes" as soon as they are aware of the movement.

How to interpret visual field defects

Bilateral field loss

Lesions from the optic chiasm to the visual cortex produce **bilateral** visual field loss and these are illustrated in Figure 2.5.

1 A hemianopia is loss of one-half of a visual field.
2 A homonymous hemianopia is loss of the temporal field of one eye and the nasal field of the other. This is due to a postchiasmatic lesion (e.g. a right homonymous hemianopia is loss of the temporal field of the right eye and the nasal field of the left eye and is due to a lesion of the left optic tract or left cerebral cortex).
3 A bitemporal hemianopia is loss of the temporal half of the visual field from both eyes. It is due to a lesion of the optic chiasm.

Unilateral field loss

Unilateral optic nerve lesions produce central field loss of the affected eye — these small areas of field loss are called scotomas.

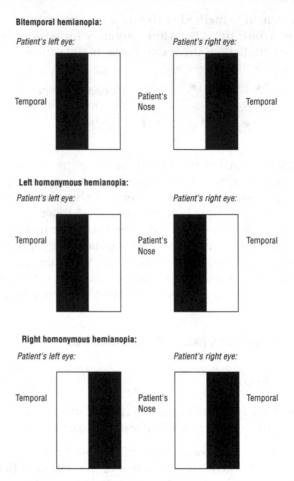

Figure 2.5 Abnormal neurological visual fields. □, Seen; ■, not seen.

Retinal and some optic nerve lesions (e.g. anterior ischaemic optic neuropathy) affect various amounts of visual field of the same eye. Unlike chiasmatic and postchiasmatic lesions, the field loss does not respect the vertical midline (the junction between the temporal and nasal fields — roughly through the centre of the pupil when testing). Glaucoma field loss can be from one or both eyes. The field loss again does not respect the vertical midline. Subtle field loss in the early stages of chronic simple glaucoma requires a sophisticated visual field analyser for detection.

Ocular movements

As outlined in Section 1, interpretation of eye movement defects can be complicated and are in the realm of the specialist. If a patient presents with symptoms of double vision (diplopia), for the non-specialist the most important thing to remember is that the examiner needs to establish whether the diplopia is monocular or binocular. To establish this from examination is quite simple:

1 The patient is asked to fix on an object in the distance, e.g. the top letter of the Snellen chart.
2 The patient's left eye is occluded (cover with your hand over a closed eyelid) and the patient is then asked whether the diplopia is still present. If the diplopia is still present, then it is monocular and due to a problem (e.g. cataract) of the right eye.
3 If the diplopia disappears, the left eye is uncovered and the right eye is then covered and the patient is asked again if diplopia is present. If the diplopia returns then the diplopia is monocular and is due to a problem in the right eye. If diplopia disappears when one eye is covered then a diagnosis of true binocular diplopia can be made.

True binocular diplopia needs same-day referral to an ophthalmologist. Patients with monocular diplopia should be advised to see their own optometrist for an up-to-date sight test. For more on diplopia see pages 105–106.

If you are testing the eye movements of the patient as part of the general examination, it can again be a very complicated and confusing process. It can however be simplified into its component parts:

1 Perform the examination in a well-lit room.
2 Use a pen-torch or climbing torch (described on page 44).
3 Sit directly in front of the patient, hold the torch just below your face, about half a metre from the patient.
4 Ask them to look directly into the light and to follow it with their **eyes** and not by moving their **head**.
5 Move the light slowly, keeping it horizontal. Start from the midline and move the light to the left, stop and return to the midline. Repeat the movement to your right.
6 Similarly, to test vertically, start at the centre and move the light upwards until the limit of the patient's gaze is found. Stop and move the light downwards until the extreme of gaze is found again.

7 Although this is simplified it will give a reasonable impression of the patient's ocular movements. Both eyes should move in complete unison and there should be no diplopia, except when the extremes of gaze are reached.

8 If there appears to be some horizontal limitation of movement of one of the eyes, the likely cause is a VIth nerve palsy. If there is vertical problem it may be a thyroid problem or an orbital blowout fracture (see appropriate topics).

Pupil reactions

How to test pupillary reactions

1 The colour of the iris and the shape and size of the pupils should be compared, preferably in a good light.

2 The pupils should then be tested for their reactions to light:
   - Perform this in a dimly lit room that is just bright enough to let you see the pupils.
   - Instruct the patient to look directly ahead and into the distance (e.g. the top letter of the 6-m Snellen chart) — this is to avoid accommodation reflexes (which themselves cause constriction of the pupil).
   - A bright pen-torch (or better a focused climbing torch such as a small Mag-lite) is then directed from below (avoiding shadow from the nose).
   - Each eye is stimulated for 3 seconds in turn to observe the pupillary reaction of the **stimulated** eye. The initial briskness and extent of any pupillary constriction is noted.
   - The swinging-light test (also known as the reactive afferent pupillary defect (RAPD) test) is then performed. The light is directed (from below) to one eye for 3 seconds and then quickly alternated between the two eyes. The afferent pupillary defect is an **extremely** important sign to look for, as if present it is invariably a sign of underlying pathology. The commonest causes are an abnormality of the optic nerve (e.g. optic neuritis or anterior ischaemic optic neuropathy) or retinal pathology (e.g. ischaemic central retinal artery occlusion and total retinal detachment).
   - Repeat the process several times, "swinging" the light from eye to eye, quickly moving your own gaze and observing only the eye that is being stimulated.

- The important observation to make here is the reaction (constriction or dilatation) of the pupil when the light is swung from the other eye. A normal reaction would be a brisk pupil constriction of the stimulated eye. During the swinging-light test, when the light is directed from the first eye to the other eye the pupil of the other eye should constrict or remain constricted (Figure 2.6).

3 The pupillary reaction for convergence is tested next. Note that if the pupillary reaction to light is **normal**, there is no need to test for reaction to convergence. Both eyes are tested together. The patient is instructed to change his/her distance gaze to a near object such as the second hand of their watch and follow it for 1 minute. Watch what happens to the pupils but do not shine a

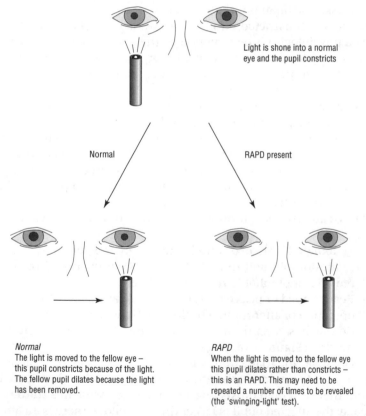

Light is shone into a normal eye and the pupil constricts

Normal

RAPD present

Normal
The light is moved to the fellow eye – this pupil constricts because of the light. The fellow pupil dilates because the light has been removed.

RAPD
When the light is moved to the fellow eye this pupil dilates rather than constricts – this is an RAPD. This may need to be repeated a number of times to be revealed (the 'swinging-light' test).

Figure 2.6 Swinging-light test for the reactive afferent pupillary defect (RAPD).

light on them. A normal reaction should be brisk constriction of both pupils as soon as the patient looks at the watch.

Thus if the pupils are equal in size and have a normal reaction to light and accommodation, it can be stated in the notes "**PERLA**" — Pupils Equally Reacting to Light and Accommodation.

Interpretation of pupillary signs

Figure 2.7 is a guide to interpreting abnormal pupil reactions and some of the more common situations are discussed below:

1 A difference in iris colour (heterochromia) suggests the possibility of inflammation, tumour or congenital Horner's syndrome. If this has not been noticed before, the patient needs to be discussed with an ophthalmologist.

2 Bilaterally constricted pupils are nowadays most commonly seen as a physiological phenomenon in the elderly. They may also be caused by local drugs such as pilocarpine (used in the treatment of glaucoma) or systemic drugs such as heroin and other morphine based compounds.

3 Extremely large pupils (mydriasis) are also usually pharmacological, e.g. patient instilling cyclopentolate drops for uveitis. Occasionally gardeners who have inadvertently brushed against the plant deadly nightshade (*Atropa belladona*) can have a temporarily dilated pupil as this plant is the source of atropine.
   Note: A dilated pupil is never a sign of coning in a patient who is **fully conscious**.

4 An irregularly shaped pupil can be due to many causes, including:
   - "Lobulated" shaped pupil caused by posterior synaechiae (adhesion of pupil to lens, Figure 2.8) in uveitis. If the eye is red and photophobic refer immediately.
   - Pear-shaped or peaked pupil in iris prolapse, e.g. after cataract operation or after trauma to the eye. If the patient is post operation or has recently had ocular trauma, immediate referral is needed (Figure 3.18, page 161).
   - Oblong pupil that extends to the periphery is an iris coloboma.

5 In Horner's syndrome the affected pupil is smaller than its fellow and there is a mild ptosis on the same side. While in a third nerve palsy the affected pupil is larger than its fellow, there is an almost complete ptosis. Both need to be referred immediately to a

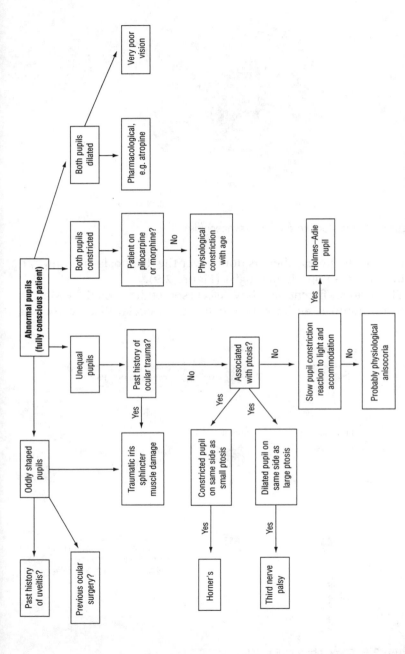

Figure 2.7 Flow diagram for assessing abnormal pupils (remember do **not** examine in a brightly lit room).

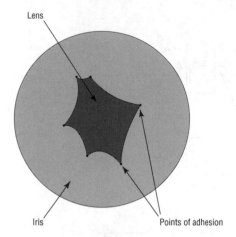

Figure 2.8 Iris stuck to the lens (synaechiae).

neurologist unless there is doubt over the diagnosis and they can be sent to an ophthalmologist (Figure 2.9).

6 The relative afferent pupillary defect (sometimes called the Marcus Gunn pupil) is an important indicator of ocular disease such as

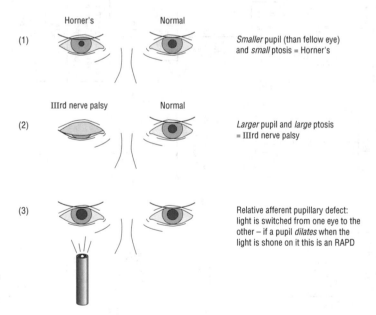

Figure 2.9 Some abnormal pupils.

optic neuropathies, ischaemic retinal disease and retinal detachment. It is discussed further in the appropriate sections on p. 38.
7 In Holmes–Adie syndrome the pupil is usually smaller than the fellow pupil and has a characteristically slow reaction to both light and convergence. These patients often need routine referral for confirmation of the diagnosis as there is no treatment.
8 Around 20% of the normal population have noticeably unequal pupil size (physiological anisocoria).

Examination of the external eye

Just like any other medical examination, the ophthalmic examination starts from the moment the patient walks into the room. Look for any obvious physical features that may be associated with underlying eye disease. Is the patient looking unwell? Is the patient in distress? Is the patient having difficulty navigating around the room?

Some ocular symptoms and signs may be relatively obvious, for example:

1 Facial features, e.g. Down's syndrome, or stature, e.g. marfanoid, are easily recognisable.
2 Photophobia.
3 Attempts by the patient to raise the eyelid to counteract a droopy upper lid (ptosis) causes an obvious wrinkling of the forehead.
4 Swelling of the eyelids in a well-looking patient may indicate a benign cause such as an acute allergic conjunctivitis whereas in an unwell-looking patient it may indicate a more serious, sight-threatening cause such as orbital cellulitis.
5 Patients with double vision sometimes cover one eye with a patch — an excellent temporary solution.
6 There are a number of syndromes which combine deafness with poor vision.
7 It is possible to get some idea of the patient's visual acuity from the way they enter the room, sit down and conduct themselves during the consultation.

Systematic examination of the external eye

As mentioned at the beginning of this section, if you are experienced in assessing eye conditions the ocular examination will be directed towards the parts of the eye that may have produced the patient's symptoms. However, for those not experienced or when no particular symptoms can be found, it may be helpful to have a systematic approach to examination of the external eye, just as it is useful to have a systematic approach to the examination of the eye in general.

It is logical to conduct the examination from front to back.

The lids and conjunctiva

The eye is a relatively small structure and this means that illumination and magnification greatly help in the examination of it. This is what makes the slit-lamp such a useful device, as it combines excellent illumination with a choice of magnification and both are aimed in the same place. Tips on using the slit-lamp are given at the end of this chapter. Unfortunately, for the beginner the slit-lamp is a rather daunting piece of equipment and partly explains why ophthalmology seems such an unapproachable specialty.

That illumination and magnification are useful is undoubtedly true, but it is not just the slit-lamp that provides this. Good illumination can be achieved with a well-lit room, a bright pen-torch or a more powerful (and expensive) pocket-sized mountaineering/climbing torch (the Mag-lite found in most camping shops is excellent). The latter has the advantage that the beam can be diffuse (useful for examining the anterior segment) or focused (useful for examining the pupils), it is more reliable and less easy to break than the pen-torch.

Magnification can be from an ordinary magnifying glass ($2\times$ to $4\times$ magnifications) or from more sophisticated binocular magnifiers such as those worn by jewellers. These have the advantage of leaving the hands free to hold the light source and to allow any manipulation that is necessary. Alternatively, it should be remembered that most practitioners already have a source of illumination and magnification — the ophthalmoscope. Turn the lens number to $+10$ (this is on the red numbers), focus on one of the patient's large conjunctival vessels, and then adjust your position back and forward when examining different parts of the external eye to keep them in focus — rather than adjusting the lens dial.

The important features to look for in the examination of the external eye are discussed below. There are more detailed descriptions in the relevant topics in Section 3.

1 **Proptosis.** This is protrusion of the globe and is a very important sign of orbital disease, e.g. thyroid eye disease or orbital cellulitis. There are two simple ways of identifying it:
   - Normally the corneoscleral junction (limbus) is covered by the upper eyelid superiorly and the lower lid inferiorly. Proptosis (globe protrusion) and retraction of the upper lid can expose the limbus.
   - Another way of determining whether there is proptosis is to stand **behind** the seated patient and look over his/her brow. Any asymmetrical protrusion of the eyeball can be seen. It is of course important to remember that the protruding eye may not be the abnormal one and that the other eye may be "sunken" (called enophthalmos), e.g. due to an orbital floor fracture.

2 **Lid position.** Look for drooping or asymmetry of position of the upper lids (ptosis) and for in-turning (entropion) or out-turning (ectropion) of the lower lids.

3 **Ocular alignment.** Generally observe the position and movements of the eyes in relation to each other — see page 37 for assessment of ocular movements.

4 **Lashes and lid margin.** This requires magnification. Look for in-turned lashes (trichiasis). Look for signs of discharge or crusting on the lids indicating conjunctivitis or blepharitis. Are there scales around the lashes like a collar (blepharitis)? Are the lid margins red and scaly (blepharitis again)? Try to look for the tear meniscus — this can normally be seen (with practice) between the posterior part of the lid margin and the conjunctiva; if missing this can be an important sign of dry eye.

5 **The conjunctiva.** A red eye (also called conjunctival hyperaemia or conjuntival injection) can be due to many causes, e.g. allergic, bacterial or viral conjunctivitis, foreign body, keratitis, uveitis or acute glaucoma. It is a non-specific sign and other symptoms and signs have to be taken into account. It is often stated that redness due to uveitis tends to be maximal around the limbus and if due to a conjunctivitis, more diffuse. In practice it is often difficult to make that distinction. Conjunctival examination is not complete until the lids are everted and the conjunctiva lining the lids (the tarsal conjunctiva) is examined — this is detailed on pages 156–157.

Conjunctival chemosis is oedema or swelling of the conjunctiva usually as part of an allergic phenomenon. It appears almost like a "jelly" coming out between the lids. It can be found in other ocular conditions, e.g. thyroid eye disease or orbital cellulitis.

The cornea

The cornea should normally be crystal clear, mirror like (e.g. you can often see a reflection of your illuminating light in it) and the iris detail is clearly visible through it. If these criteria do not hold then it is necessary to find out why.

Specifically look for:

1 **Foreign bodies.** These are usually seen as small black or brown spots on the surface of the cornea.
2 **Discrete corneal opacities.** Discrete white/yellow corneal opacities in the presence of an injected (i.e. red) eye suggest active corneal inflammation (keratitis). Opacities in the presence of a white (i.e. un-inflamed) eye suggest a previous episode of keratitis or an old injury.
3 **Diffuse corneal opacities.** A diffuse, hazy cornea (dull, with no light reflection) with a hazy view of the iris may be due to corneal oedema, extensive keratitis or severe chemical burns.
4 **Corneal endothelium.** This cannot be seen without high magnification, but it can sometimes be highlighted by large inflammatory deposits (keratic precipitates) sticking to it. They are a sign of intraocular inflammation, usually acute anterior uveitis.
5 **Corneal sensation.** Certain conditions can reduce corneal sensation and are an important sign of these diseases:
   - Sensation can be tested with a wisp of cotton twisted to form a point.
   - The patient is instructed to look straight ahead, and the cotton wisp is brought near the eye from the temporal side and touched gently on the cornea.
   - Reflex closure of the eyelids occurs with normal innervation.
   - Avoid touching the eyelashes or lid margin as this also provokes reflex closure of the eyelids.
   - Corneal sensation should be compared to the other eye by asking the patient if there is any difference in sensation.
   - Corneal sensation testing is only valid prior to instillation of anaesthetic drops to the eye.
   - Corneal sensation can be reduced in herpes simplex keratitis, herpes zoster ophthalmicus cerebellopontine angle tumours and contact lens wearers.

Using fluorescein

Fluorescein is a dye with the useful property of being able to absorb one wavelength of light and emit a different one, i.e. it fluoresces. This fluorescence only occurs if a blue light is shone at the fluorescein — this is why most pen-torches have a small blue cap that fits over the end of them and these should be used whenever fluorescein is used. A Woods light, which is usually used by dermatologists, can be very useful if available. It emits the appropriate blue light and often has a magnifier with it. It can be especially useful in children where the fluorescein drops are instilled, the room lights switched off and the Woods light switched on, the fluorescein then lights up like a beacon.

Fluorescein drops are essential for the diagnosis of most corneal disorders, especially those in which the epithelium has been damaged, e.g. corneal abrasions or herpes simplex infection. The reason fluorescein shows up epithelial damage so well is because of a difference in concentration between areas on the cornea where epithelial cells are present and where they are absent. If a corneal abrasion is present, fluorescein will collect in the base of it and form a thicker layer of stain than that on the surrounding, normal, epithelium. When the blue light is switched on the area with the greater amount of stain fluoresces more and is immediately obvious.

Fluorescein drops come in single-use plastic droppers (called minims) and the appropriate concentration for looking for epithelial changes is 2%. Also available are fluorescein-impregnated paper strips which need to be wetted with sterile water or saline (**not** tap water) and are then placed in the lower fornix (for 1–2 seconds) — with the lower lid being pulled down and the patient looking up.

Contact lenses must be removed before fluorescein is instilled as it can stain them — they should not be replaced for at least 20 minutes.

The anterior chamber

After examining the cornea it is important to look behind it into the anterior chamber (AC). The AC is a three-dimensional space but without binocular magnification it will not be perceived as such. The more obvious abnormalities of the AC include:

1 **Hyphaema.** This is blood in the anterior chamber that has settled — like sand that has passed through an egg-timer. It usually occurs after blunt trauma to the eye (Figure 3.17, p. 161).
2 **Hypopyon.** This is similar to a hyphaema but consists of inflammatory cells rather than red blood cells and is therefore white rather than red.
3 **Fibrin.** In some types of uveitis thin white strands of fibrin can be seen in the AC and they are a marker of inflammation. Using the high magnification of the slit-lamp it is possible to see individual cells within the AC, but this takes quite a lot of practice.

Examination of the iris and pupil are discussed on page 38. The lens can be examined using the ophthalmoscope and this is discussed below.

Optic disc and retina

The posterior part of the eye (also called the ocular fundus) containing the retina, choroid, optic disc, macula and fovea cannot be viewed without using condensing lenses and illumination. There are three ways of achieving this:

1 Direct ophthalmoscopy — this is the normal hand-held ophthalmoscope
2 The slit-lamp with specially adapted lenses — this is described at the end of the section.
3 Indirect ophthalmoscopy.

The latter two methods are mainly used in specialist settings and will only be briefly discussed. The direct ophthalmoscope is used worldwide by almost all medical practitioners and it is vital to know how to use it.

Direct ophthalmoscopy

This provides an upright image, magnified to about 15 times. If only the optic disc and macular area are to be examined and the pupils are reasonably well dilated no pupillary dilatation may be required. If, however, the pupils are small or a larger area needs to be viewed the pupils are dilated — the method for doing this and precautions to take are discussed at the end of this section (see page 62).

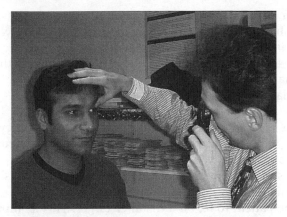

Figure 2.10 (a) Note: fingers and palm hold head still. Thumbs hold lid open. Red reflex checked at arm's length.

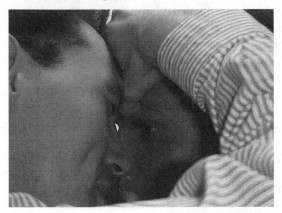

Figure 2.10 (b) Note: Use the first joint of your thumb as an indicator of where your eyebrow should rest. Avoid obscuring the patient's other eye or fixation will be lost.

Described below is a method of approaching the ophthalmoscope that after some practice will consistently allow viewing of the ocular fundus (optic nerve, disc, macula). Figure 2.10 illustrates some of the steps:

1 Before you start check if the ophthalmoscope is working and bring the appropriate lens up before you turn the lights off! Switch on the ophthalmoscope light to maximum; if it does not form a bright spot of light on your hand change the batteries. Set all figures on the numbered dials on the front to "0".

2 If your ophthalmoscope has coloured filters or different spot sizes/shapes forget about them. Use the ordinary white light and with the ophthalmoscope switched on, turn the spot size to the smallest spot, then use ONE size larger than this.

3 Ophthalmoscopic examination should be performed in a dimly lit or dark room.

4 Forget all about your refraction and the patient's. Take your glasses off and take the patient's glasses off — they only get in the way. If you or the patient have contact lenses don't worry about it, leave them in.

5 Make sure the patient is comfortable and that he/she is at a convenient height for you to examine.

6 Ask the patient to fix on a distance target. This is important, do not vaguely say "look into the distance" but choose a specific object and tell the patient to keep staring at it and to tell you if you get between them and the target. The patient should not look into the light of the ophthalmoscope until you tell them to.

7 Although not vital, when you are examining the right eye choose a target that is slightly to the patient's left and vice-versa for the other eye. This means you are less likely to block the patient's view of the target and it actually makes the optic disc easier to find.

8 Although not popular it is much better to examine the patient's right eye with the ophthalmoscope held in your right hand using your right eye and the patient's left eye with the ophthalmoscope in your left hand and using your left eye. This does take some practice but the alternative involves blocking the patient's view at best and almost kissing the patient at worst!

9 Always hold the ophthalmoscope so that your index finger is on the lens dial but keep the dial on "0" for the time being.

10 Whichever hand you are using to hold the ophthalmoscope, place the palm of your other hand on the forehead of the patient above the eye you are about to examine. The position of your thumb is vital, it should be resting gently on the patient's upper lid. This means the rest of your fingers are splayed across the patient's forehead and act to keep the head still (see Figure 2.10(a)).

11 You are using your thumb for two things. Firstly to keep the patient's upper eyelid open and secondly as a marker for where your forehead should be (Figure 2.10(b)). The mistake most people make with the ophthalmoscope is to be too far away from the eye and this is why you either get no view or a distant, fleeting image of the disc. Placing your forehead (just

above your eyebrow) on your thumb means the ophthalmoscope is near enough for a good view but not too near.

12 Before having a close look, stand looking through your ophthalmoscope at arm's length from the patient (you already have your hand on the patient's forehead (Figure 2.10(a))). Shine the light into the pupil until you see a red/orange glow coming from the pupil. This is the red reflex and represents light entering the eye and being reflected back again. Thus if there is any opacity in the cornea, lens or vitreous the light will not be reflected back again and a dark area will be seen. The commonest cause for this is opacities in the lens (cataract).

13 If there is no red reflex then you will not get a view of the fundus.

14 Once the red reflex has been seen, move your head so that it takes up position on your thumb as described above. This should immediately give you a view of the retina and optic disc — do not worry if, in young patients, you appear to be getting a lot of reflections from the retinal surface, this is quite normal. Use the yellow optic disc as a reference point — it is relatively easy to find and is an important landmark.

15 In all likelihood the disc will be out of focus because of your or the patient's refractive error and you need to bring up the appropriate lens in the ophthalmoscope. **Do not** do this by **looking** at the numbers but (while maintaining you position) simply turn the lens dial with your index finger — if the disc becomes more blurry then turn the dial in the opposite direction until the disc comes into sharp focus.

16 Move your head and the ophthalmoscope to look around the posterior pole. Last of all, ask the patient to look directly into the ophthalmoscope light — you will then automatically be looking at the macula and fovea. The fovea, especially in young people, can be seen as a tiny light in the centre of the retina — this is known as the foveal reflex.

It is important to remember that you are only seeing a small part of the retina with the direct ophthalmoscope. It is very useful for the posterior pole but cannot examine the peripheral retina and for conditions such as retinal detachment specialist equipment is required. The direct ophthalmoscope is uniocular and therefore it can be difficult to assess if lesions are raised or not.

When drawing what you see through the ophthalmoscope remember that the macula/fovea is temporal to the disc.

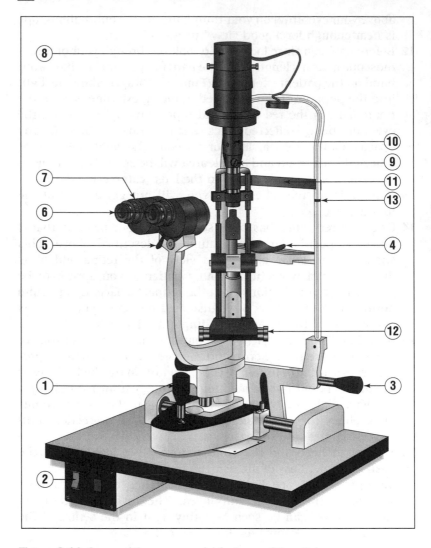

Figure 2.11 Some of the more useful features of the slit-lamp.

Parts of slit-lamp
1 Control lever for horizontal (by twisting) and vertical (by pushing) adjustment
2 Switch for on/off and adjustment of illumination level (varies between manufacturers, but always aim to examine the patient at the lowest illumination possible)
3 Handles for patient to grip (cont'd on following page)

Indirect ophthalmoscopy

This is an ophthalmoscope which you wear on the head and requires a condensing lens (usually +20 dioptre) held in one hand. It has the advantage that it is binocular and gives an excellent view of the peripheral retina, especially if the free hand is used to depress the sclera.

The disadvantage of the ophthalmoscope is that it takes a lot of practice to become familiar with, it is expensive and the image it gives is inverted and laterally transposed.

Using the slit-lamp

The slit-lamp is essentially a binocular microscope mounted on a table, i.e. it is simply a convenient way of combining magnification with illumination. The focal distance is short so that the patient is near enough to allow the examiner to be able to reach the eye. When first encountered the slit-lamp appears to be a complex piece of equipment but a few basics rules can make it much easier to use (see overleaf):

4   Chin rest
5   Lever for changing low to high magnification
6   Eye-pieces
7   Rings for setting eye-pieces (like binoculars the focus is adjusted until the image is clear)
8   Cover for bulb
9   Control for rotation of slit and varying the slit length (sometimes the blue light is put on with this)
10 Lever for varying colour of light (the blue light is used to highlight fluorescein)
11 Band for forehead. It is extremely important that the patient has his/her head against this throughout the examination firstly so that the eye remains in focus and secondly to prevent them moving forward onto the needle when a foreign body is being removed
12 Knob for controlling the width of the slit (hence increasing or decreasing the amount of light)
13 Mark on metal upright. This indicates the approximate level that the patient's eyes should be at when being examined — the chin rest can usually be moved up and down to get the eyes to this level

1 If you have not used a slit-lamp before it is worth having a fiddle with the slit-lamp before seeing a patient with it — Figure 2.11 highlights some of the more useful features.

2 Switching the slit-lamp on can sometimes be a puzzle in itself: (numbers relate to Figure 2.11)
   – Check it is plugged in and the socket is switched on.
   – Turn the off/on switch ② usually located just under the table-top on the left side of the lamp. If the switch is a dial with a choice of positions only turn it one turn.
   – If the light does not come on (hold your hand in front of the illumination column to check) turn the knob at the base of the illumination column ⑫ right round until the light appears.
   – If the light still does not appear or the light is either blue or green, flick switch ⑩ as far left as it will go.
   – If the light still has not come on then seek help, it may be the bulb (situated at the very top of the illumination column ⑧) that has blown.

3 Once you have switched it on, ask a colleague if you can look at his/her eyes. Position both yourself and the colleague comfortably, with the colleague's chin in the chin rest ④ without having to stretch his/her neck. This is achieved by adjusting the height of the slit-lamp table, usually via a lever found underneath the centre of the table or in older lamps by turning a wheel situated near the base of the table. Do not adjust the height of the slit-lamp when the subject has the chin in the chin rest, as it can move down suddenly.

4 Once the subject has his/her chin rested comfortably on the chin-rest, ask him/her to push their forehead up against the horizontal plastic bar ⑪.

5 On your side of the lamp, adjust the binocular eye-pieces ⑥ so that they are on "0" — just like an ordinary pair of binoculars. Look down the eye-pieces and adjust them so that you can see down both eye-pieces — again just like a pair of binoculars. If you wear glasses you can wear them to look down the eye-pieces or if you know your refractive error you can adjust this on the eye-pieces and remove your glasses. Patients are never examined with their glasses on.

6 During the eye examination, focusing is obtained by moving the whole magnification column back and forward, often with a centrally placed joystick ①. If inexperienced in this it can take some practice to get used to the more subtle movement required. The whole column is moved up and down either by turning

the joystick or a small wheel at the base of the magnification column.

7 Illumination can be varied during the examination by turning the knob at the base of the illumination column ⑫ and this gradually changes the shape of the light beam from large and diffuse to a thin slit (hence the name slit-lamp). At the start of the examination use diffuse light but make sure it is not too bright.

8 Using the slip-lamp is very like using a low magnification laboratory microscope. Using a general illumination (wide-opened slit) a magnified image of the eye structures (conjunctiva, cornea, anterior chamber, iris and lens) can be viewed. A slit-beam is used to give depth to structures like the cornea (e.g. a corneal abscess can be seen within the depth of the corneal stroma). If using fluorescein, the blue light is switched on using the lever ⑨ or ⑩.

9 The retina can only be seen by using various kinds of accessory lenses (e.g. 90-dioptre lens). This requires some practice and is generally not used by the primary practitioner.

Examination in difficult circumstances

The information under the following headings provides some tips for examining the eyes in less than ideal circumstances. Not only can it be useful to use different examination techniques but also to be aware of the limitations to the information you are likely to gain in these circumstances.

Examining the child

General inspection

How thorough an examination can be conducted very much depends on the age of the child but can be influenced by your approach to the child and the child's previous experiences. The first step should always be "hands-off". While taking the history from the parents allow the child to roam around the room to become familiarised with it. Once your attention turns to the child spend a few minutes observing his/her behaviour — this can often give vital clues to the diagnosis:

1 Is the child's visual behaviour normal, i.e. is he/she walking into large objects in the room; is he/she seeing and picking up small toys/objects?
2 Is the child in pain — holding the eye closed with the hand, e.g. corneal abrasion?
3 Is the child unwell, e.g. orbital cellulitis?
4 Is the child avoiding the light, e.g. keratitis, uveitis or congenital glaucoma?

Visual function

It is essential to make an attempt to assess the child's vision — again, this will obviously depend on the age of the child. Many children from 6 years onwards will be able to read the Snellen chart (remember to do this one eye at a time). It is worth remembering that children with amblyopic eyes can read single letters much better than rows of letters. If the child does not know their letters particularly well, print some of the letters on a piece of paper, ask the child to hold the sheet and point to some of the Snellen chart letters, asking the child to point to the same letters. It is better to use relatively simple letters such as "O" and "X". This technique can also be used for those who are illiterate or who do not know the English alphabet.

With even younger children, without specialist equipment it is difficult to measure their visual acuity, but it is not difficult to get some idea of their visual function. General visual function can be assessed by a few methods and the examiner can use a combination of these:

1 The child's fixation (e.g. to the mother's face) can be observed to determine the child's "visual alertness".
2 For very young children, a pen-torch can be used to test the fixation. It can be switched on and off to attract the child's attention and then moved from side to side and up and down to see if the child follows it.
3 For those over 6 months, brightly coloured objects or toys that do not make any sound can also be used. The object can be brought into the view of the child from behind the child to see if the child fixates to the object. Once the child's attention is obtained cover each eye in turn and make sure each eye follows the object. It is also worth noting the child's reaction to occlusion of the eye. If the child objects to one eye being covered but not the other,

this can sometimes suggest that the vision in the eye they did **not** object to being covered is poor.

4 For those over 1 year "hundreds and thousands" cake decorations are a useful test of visual function. They are scattered in the palm of the examiner or parent's hand and if the child sees them he/she will usually try to pick them up. Test with both eyes open initially and then one eye at a time. They equate to around 6/18 Snellen vision.

If there is **any** question of a child's vision being impaired, the child must be referred to an orthoptist or ophthalmologist.

Squints

If a parent presents with a child and feels (or someone else, e.g. grandmother, nursery) the child is squinting (i.e. the eyes are not aligned, **not** that the eyelids are closed in bright light) then the child must be referred to an orthoptist/ophthalmologist for full assessment, refraction and fundoscopy.

Probably the most important element of the examination in these circumstances is to look for a red reflex — if a child does not have a red reflex or it is different between the two eyes they must be referred immediately.

The simplest way of looking for a squint in a child is to sit in front of them with a pen-torch, shine it at them and ask them to keep looking at it. Look for an obvious squint, if you can see one, cover each eye slowly in turn and watch what movement the eye makes when it is uncovered. The squint is in the opposite direction to the movement the eye makes when it is uncovered.

Finally, ask the child to keep staring at the light and move it left to right and up and down — normally both eyes move to the extremes of gaze, if they do not then think of a muscle palsy and refer immediately.

External eye examination

Probably one of the commonest presentations of children is with a sticky eye and examination of the external eye is necessary. Again, observing the child in a well-lit room can provide a great deal of information. A pen-torch can be used for more directed illumination — it is often difficult to use a magnifier with children as they tend to feel easily crowded and move around a great deal. For any child with a red or sore eye try look for certain features:

1 Bilateral, crusty, sticky lids strongly suggest infective conjunctivitis.
2 Examine the cornea for foreign bodies.
3 Look at the cornea and see how it reflects your light, it should be shiny. If it is dull or hazy refer immediately.
4 If possible gently evert the upper eyelid to exclude any subtarsal foreign bodies. This may require topical anaesthetic — g.proxymetacaine is best as it is minimally stinging, otherwise use g.benoxinate.
5 Always try to stain the cornea with 2% fluorescein drops as corneal abrasions are common in children. Using the Wood's light for this can be very helpful (see below).
6 Look for a red reflex.

A child with a red eye should have a thorough eye examination and if necessary be wrapped in a blanket to prevent him/her from using their hands to interfere with the examination. This procedure is very distressing to the child and should be done with the help of the parents. A good illumination is required to examine the clarity of the cornea and exclude any corneal foreign bodies. The upper eyelid is everted to exclude any subtarsal foreign bodies. The cornea is stained with fluorescein drops and the cornea examined for any epithelial defect.

A Woods light can be very useful for examining children (or adults). It is an illuminated magnifier (useful in itself for examining the eye) and also has a blue light source. 2% Fluorescein can be instilled into the eye, the Woods light switched on and the room lights off. When the child opens their eyes (this may take some time) any abrasion will be spontaneously obvious.

The posterior pole

It is often difficult to examine the retina in children without specialist equipment. The direct ophthalmoscope is very difficult to use — it can appear threatening to children and requires them to keep their eye still. If a child needs a retinal examination they should be referred the same day.

What must **always** be done with the direct ophthalmoscope is to look for a red reflex and this must be documented. Although rare, retinoblastoma can present with a squint — loss of the red reflex is an important sign of this and same-day ophthalmic referral is necessary.

Examining the neonate

The eyes of the newborn are examined by the non-ophthalmologist in two common situations:

1 **Ophthalmia neonatorum** — i.e. conjunctivitis within the first month of life. Check that the cornea is clear, take swabs for bacteria and chlamydia. This needs immediate referral to an ophthalmologist or paediatrician.
2 **Routine postnatal red reflex check** — this is done with the direct ophthalmoscope in a dimly lit room. The baby should be at roughly two-thirds of your arm's length away. If the baby is asleep get someone to gently open the baby's lids. If the baby is screwing their eyes tightly shut because they are crying ask the mother to feed the baby and check for the red reflex during this. The presence of the red reflex is important, if there are any doubts contact an ophthalmologist.

It is generally not necessary to dilate the neonate's pupil to get the red reflex but if this cannot be avoided use cyclopentolate 0.5% both eyes. Phenylephrine 2.5% (one drop only) can also be used if the pupil is not dilating.

Examining the demented patient

Like the child, the demented patient will not complain of visual symptoms. However this means that they can have significant visual pathology without anyone being aware — this is important as any sensory deprivation is going to add to their dementia. Ask any carers or relatives how much they feel the patient can see — this can give very important clues as to visual performance.

Try to make a gross assessment of the vision by covering one eye at a time and moving your hand in the four quadrants of the visual field (supra- and infero- nasal and temporal). If the patient responds this means that they can see your hand, they have a grossly normal visual field and that their eye movements are grossly normal.

Examine the outer eye with a torch and magnifier, direct ophthalmoscope or the slit-lamp and look for the features of external eye disease discussed above. Check for an RAPD (see page 38).

Dilate the pupil with g.tropicamide 1% and g.phenylephrine 2.5% (do not use 10%, these patients are often quite frail) and check the red reflex carefully; these patients often have cataract. Examine the back of the eye looking for optic nerve and macular (usually ARMD) disease.

Examining the bed-ridden patient

To examine the bed-ridden patient, it is only possible to use equipment that is portable:

1 The reduced Snellen chart (see page 29) or a near reading chart can be used at the bedside. If these are not available newsprint is roughly equivalent to N8. Do not forget that the patient should use reading glasses if they normally do — if they did not bring them or lost them it is perfectly good to borrow someone else's, although they must be reading glasses only, not bifocals.
2 A pen-torch, a blue filter, fluorescein eye drops and a magnifying glass can be used in the normal manner (described earlier).
3 Eye movements and pupil reactions can usually be examined at the bedside.
4 Pupils can be dilated, but take care that this does not interfere with any neurological monitoring.

Examining the ventilated patient

It is not uncommon for ventilated patients to have ophthalmic problems related to their underlying problem or the ventilation itself:

1 **Corneal exposure.** This occurs because of inadequate corneal protection in the sedated patient. Prevention is better than cure and it is important to make sure that the lids are covering the cornea (e.g. taping the lids shut) or use artificial methods to keep the cornea lubricated (e.g. wet swabs, bubble chambers, Occ. Simplex qds). If a corneal abrasion forms the eye becomes very injected — chronically exposed eyes may be mildly injected,

but a relatively sudden increase in redness must be treated with caution. Fluorescein 2% and a blue light will show any abrasion. Prescribe Occ. chloramphenicol 2 hourly to the affected eye and ask for an ophthalmologist to review.

2 **Microbial keratitis**. This can occur secondary to a corneal abrasion or prolonged epithelial abnormalities due to drying. It also presents with a sudden increase in injection of the eye and on examining the cornea a white opacity can be seen. Do not prescribe antibiotics but contact the on-call ophthalmologist.

3 **Conjunctival chemosis**. This is an uncommon and poorly recognised feature of patients on ventilators. It is relatively quick and presents as a "jelly" coming out of the eye — the jelly is the swollen conjunctiva. It settles spontaneously, but the conjunctiva needs protection from drying. Prescribe Occ. chloramphenicol qds and cover the affected eye with saline-soaked pads until the conjunctiva has resumed its normal position.

4 **Optic disc swelling**. This can occur secondary to raised intracranial pressure (papilloedema), when it is bilateral, or as a result of direct damage to the optic canal and subsequent pressure on the optic nerve, when it is usually unilateral. To detect optic canal fracture needs a high index of suspicion and an awareness that the condition exists. Typical features are:
 – Significant head injury — especially to the brow and forehead.
 – Optic disc swelling but an otherwise normal retina.
 – An RAPD.
 CT scanning is the investigation of choice looking at the optic canal in detail. Neurosurgical consultation is also required — if there is an obvious optic nerve sheath haematoma it needs to be decompressed, otherwise IV steroid may be of benefit.

5 **Hyphaema**. Spontaneous hyphaemas (visible blood in the anterior chamber (Figure 3.17, page 161)) can be seen as part of the overall trauma, can occur because of accidental trauma to the eye in the unconscious patient or sometimes in coronary care units after thrombolysis. The haemorrhage itself is not harmful and it will be absorbed spontaneously but there is a danger that it will cause the intraocular pressure (IOP) to rise. Ophthalmic opinion and monitoring of IOP are required.

6 **Retinal/vitreous haemorrhages**. These can occur because of the original trauma, because of a sudden increase in intracranial pressure, secondary to thrombolysis or after CPR (due to chest compression). They generally resolve spontaneously but need ophthalmic observation. Similarly, retinal fat emboli (small

yellowy lesions in the retinal vessels) usually from fracture of long bones tend to resolve spontaneously.

Dilating the pupil

Pupil dilation is an area that causes some concern to non-ophthalmologists — the worry being that you will precipitate closed angle glaucoma. In fact this is an unlikely occurrence and it is usually true that it was going to occur in the near future anyway. It is really the apparent cause and effect relationship that makes it seem so bad. It is much more likely that serious harm will come to the patient with unrecognised retinal pathology, e.g. diabetic retinopathy or retinal detachment, than from a quickly recognised and treated closed angle episode.

However, before dilating anyone it is worth asking them:

1 Have you ever been told you should not have your pupil dilated — some patient's with narrow drainage angles (and who do not have a peripheral iridectomy: Figure 2.12) are told this by their ophthalmologists.
2 Patients who have symptoms of intermittent angle closure, i.e. attacks of haloes/rainbows around lights, blurred vision or ocular pain in the evenings should not be dilated and should be discussed immediately with the on-call ophthalmologist.

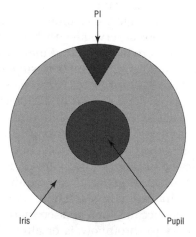

Figure 2.12 Peripheral iridectomy (PI). The treatment for angle closure glaucoma.

If a patient is known to have narrow angles and has had a peripheral iridectomy (PI) (Figure 2.12), it is safe to dilate their pupils. A similar principle holds for those systemic medications (usually anticholinergics, e.g. antidepressants) that state in their contraindications "not to be given to patients with glaucoma" — this is usually narrow angle glaucoma and if the patient has this type and not had a PI then this contraindication holds. If they have any other sort of glaucoma such as primary open angle, then this will not be affected by the medication.

For most purposes dilation with g.tropicamide 1% is safe and adequate to get a view of the disc and macula area. If greater dilation is needed use g.phenylephrine, but it is important to be aware that in certain patients it should be used with care (see page 177).

Other cautions with pupil dilation:

1 Always check pupil responses before dilating.
2 If a patient is going to require neurological monitoring check with ward staff before dilating
3 When referring a patient who has been dilated do not forget to inform the unit that the patient is going to be referred to of this fact.
4 Visual acuity is affected in a variable manner after dilation, as a rule patients should not drive until the effects have completely worn off (can take 3 or 4 hours). It is worth informing the patient of this prior to dilation.

Using topical anaesthetic

Topical anaesthetics play a vital role in ophthalmic examination and procedures, however they should be used with care:

1 After using topical anaesthetic corneal sensation is temporarily reduced, the eye can be rubbed or foreign bodies can enter the eye and cause damage without symptoms. Warn the patient of this and ask him/her to wait for 30 minutes before going outside — if the patient is being padded anyway this will protect the eye.
2 Do not replace contact lenses for at least 30 minutes.
3 **Never** use topical anaesthetics to treat an eye condition, e.g. abrasion. Patients will ask for this because of the relief they get from them, but in fact they are toxic to the epithelium and will actually make things worse.

Section 3
What you should do

This section is intended as a guide to what to do with the patient once the diagnosis has been made. Most of the commonly encountered eye conditions will be in this section.

Most topics contain a section on the typical presenting features of the disorder, although in some sections this approach is inappropriate. This is followed by an outline of the basic principles of treatment and finally a description of what needs to be done.

Some topics are not condition based but are intended to give a quick overview for the non-ophthalmologists of important conditions and situations.

The section is divided into further sections based mainly on the typical presenting symptoms of the various conditions. It is important to remember that many of the conditions can present in more than one way and the topics should be used in conjunction with Sections 1 and 2.

N.B. Main referral priorities indicated in the text:
Immediate referral Means the opthalmologist should be
        contacted by telephone so that the patient can be seen
        immediately
Same-day referral Seen within 24 hours
Routine referral Means sending a letter to outpatients

Decreased vision without pain

Anterior ischaemic optic neuropathy (AION)

Typical presentation

Anterior ischaemic optic neuropathy is infarction of the optic disc.
This may be secondary to arteritic processes (i.e. temporal arteritis)
or non-arteritic. The non-arteritic type can be idiopathic, but
more commonly occurs in patient with hypertension, diabetes or
atherosclerosis. It can also be seen in patients who have suffered
hypovolaemic blood loss or who have had a sudden drop in their
blood pressure.

AION presents with sudden loss of vision in one eye often on
waking. There is no associated pain unless the patient has the
headache of temporal arteritis. Dilation of the pupils reveals a
swollen optic disc, often with haemorrhages and cotton-wool
spots on it.

The usual age group is around 60–65 years of age for the non-
arteritic type and 70–75 years for the arteritic type.

Principles of treatment

1 Look for the signs and symptoms of temporal arteritis — always
  check the ESR
2 For the non-arteritic type of AION there is no treatment but the
  patient needs same day referral for a definitive diagnosis.
3 If the patient has symptoms or signs of temporal arteritis or the
  ESR is very high, immediate treatment with steroids is needed
  to prevent infarction of the fellow optic nerve.
4 The patient with non-arteritic AION also has a significant long
  term risk of sustaining an AION in the fellow eye and risk
  factors must be addressed.

How and what to do

1 Question the patient carefully regarding signs and symptoms of
  temporal arteritis (see page 17 for these).

2 Check the visual acuity — this can be variable but tends to be markedly reduced. In the non-arteritic type it is often 6/60 or CFS. In the artertic type the visual loss is usually even more profound PL or NPL.

3 Test for an RAPD. This will be present unless the patient has had a previous AION in the fellow eye.

4 Check the colour vision (especially if the diagnosis is uncertain) although in AION the vision is usually too poor for the patient to see the test plate.

5 Dilate both pupils with tropicamide 1%. The disc changes are usually obvious — the disc margins cannot be seen and the disc looks swollen. Usually there are haemorrhages and cotton-wool spots on the disc. If there are haemorrhages more peripherally think of central retinal vein occlusion.

6 The ESR **must** be checked whatever the findings. The normal ranges for ESR are given on page 70.

7 Management:
   - The patient needs immediate referral to eye casualty. Inform the referral doctor of important past medical history and drugs — ask for the ESR to be phoned through.
   - If the patient has symptoms or signs of temporal arteritis or an ESR above 50 mm/hr steroids are required.
   - When the diagnosis of temporal arteritis is suspected treatment must begin immediately (see page 70).
   - For non-ischaemic AION the risk to the fellow eye is lower than in the arteritic type, but remains significant at around 40% over 10 years (this varies depending on other risk factors). Once this diagnosis has been made, look at patient risk factors such as smoking, hyperlipidaemia, anaemia and diabetic control.

Amaurosis fugax (visual transient ischaemic attacks)

Typical presentation

Patients typically complain of sudden loss of vision lasting for a few minutes (although it can last longer) that returns completely to normal afterwards. It may have happened previously and is usually unilateral. By the time the patient is seen there are usually no ocular signs.

Principles of treatment

The underlying pathology is a temporary interruption to the blood supply of the retina. The most common cause is an embolus from the carotid artery, heart or aorta that becomes lodged in the retina circulation. Although no ocular treatment is required full cardiovascular work-up is necessary.

How and what to do

1 When taking the history, remember there are other causes of intermittent loss of vision including:
  – temporal arteritis
  – migraine
  – impending central retinal vein occlusion
  – papilloedema
  – acute closed angle glaucoma.
2 Ocular examination should include visual acuity, pupillary defects and dilated fundoscopy.
3 A thorough medical examination is important, especially examining for bruits in the carotid circulation and the heart and checking the pulse for atrial fibrillation. Do not forget to palpate the temporal arteries.
4 Take blood for an urgent ESR and for FBC, glucose and lipids.
5 Start the patient on aspirin 75 mg/day (if there are no contra-indications).
6 Advise the patient to stop smoking.
7 Refer the patient by telephone to a cardiologist for an urgent outpatient appointment.

Central retinal artery occlusion (CRAO)

Typical presentation

The patient is over 60 years of age and has noticed a sudden loss of vision in one eye. There are no antecedent symptoms (unless they have been getting warning TIAs) and the visual loss is painless (**important exception** to this is CRAO secondary to temporal arteritis). Commonly the patient notices the visual loss first thing in the morning. The patient often has other markers of athero-sclerosis.

Important signs that help make the diagnosis are a profound loss in vision, e.g. counting fingers, light perception. The presence of an afferent pupillary defect and the presence an embolus in one of the retinal vessels. The optic disc should not be swollen or have sur-rounding haemorrhages, as this would indicate an AION (which shares many of the same features).

Principles of treatment

1 CRAO is caused by a sudden blockage of the central retinal artery leading to retinal ischaemia. This may be caused by carotid or cardiac emboli, haemorrhage into an atheromatous plaque or because of inflammation in the arterial wall.
2 Treatment of the blockage itself is controversial as the time taken for irreversible retinal ischaemia to occur is not known and will differ depending on the amount of retina that has become ischae-mic. Spontaneous recovery is common, making evaluation of treatment difficult.
3 It is important to be aware that CRAO is usually associated with systemic disease, that cardiovascular disease is the major cause of death and that cerebrovascular disease is the major cause of morbidity in these patients.

How and what to do

Because of the variation in response to ischaemia, many ophthal-mologists would attempt treatment to try to reverse the ischaemia if the patient presents within 24 hours of the onset of symptoms. CRAO can present in one of three ways:

1 Visual loss for less than 24 hours.
2 Visual loss for more than 24 hours.
3 Secondary to temporal arteritis.

Even though visual recovery is very unlikely if symptoms are present for longer than 24 hours, most ophthalmologists would suggest that non-invasive treatment should be attempted up to 24 hours after onset of symptoms. The patient will often feel psychologically better if some form of treatment is tried. Before you start any treatment you must tell the patient that the prognosis for visual recovery is poor.

1 Presentation within 24 hours:
 – Refer the patient to eye casualty by telephone.
 – Take blood for an urgent ESR and ask the laboratory to ring both yourself and the eye department with the result as soon as available.
 – If the history or examination is consistent with temporal arteritis give 200–300 mg IV hydrocortisone or 500 mg–1 g IV methyl prednisolone (given slowly over 15 min).
 – If it is not, give the patient 300 mg aspirin (unless contra-indicated). If the patient usually takes GTN for angina it will do no harm to take a dose and this may have a beneficial effect on the central artery.
 – Once the patient is seen in eye casualty other methods of improving the ocular blood flow may be attempted.

2 Presentation over 24 hours:
 – Take blood for an urgent ESR.
 – There is no treatment for the eye at this stage and management is to prevent other cardiovascular events including CRAO of the fellow eye.
 – A complete cardiovascular evaluation is needed, including BP, carotids, and bloods.
 – The patient needs an urgent Doppler ultrasound and an urgent referral to the vascular surgeons. Until the appointment, start aspirin 75 mg daily.

3 Temporal arteritis:
 – For signs and symptoms see page 17. If these lead you to believe that temporal arteritis underlies CRAO than take an urgent ESR but begin treatment with steroids as described above.
 – A guide for a raised ESR is $0.5 \times$ age in men and $0.5 \times$ age + 10 in women. However the result of the ESR must be taken in the context of the other findings.
 – It is not unusual in cases of temporal arteritis for the ESR to be within the normal range.
 – The patient needs **immediate** referral to an ophthalmologist.

Posterior vitreous detachment (PVD) and retinal detachment (RD)

Typical presentation

Patients usually complain of a sudden onset of "spiders, cobwebs or floaters" in their visual axis. They may experience flashing lights "like little bits of lightning". They may associate the onset of symptoms with sudden physical activity such as sneezing or trauma. These symptoms indicate a collapse/liquefaction of the vitreous, i.e. posterior vitreous detachment or PVD.

A partial or complete loss of vision, usually after the onset of the above symptoms, may indicate that the retina has detached.

Principles of treatment

1 If a patient presents with a recent onset or change in floaters or flashing lights described above then refer the patient the same day to an ophthalmologist.
2 PVDs do not need treatment and the floaters usually settle with time. The treatment of retinal detachment is operative.
3 Because someone has had previous retinal surgery does not mean that they cannot have a further retinal detachment and these patients also need to be referred.

How and what to do

1 Floaters are a specific symptom and indicate changes in the vitreous. They are extremely common especially in myopes, The important feature in the history is the **change** in floaters — this always requires ophthalmic assessment.
2 When referring the patient it is helpful for the ophthalmologist to know:
   – The visual acuity — a reduced visual acuity may indicate that the retinal detachment (RD) has involved the macula.
   – If there is an afferent pupillary defect.
   – The patient's past medical and drug history — if they have an RD the only treatment is operative. If the retina is torn but not

detached, laser is used to seal the hole and prevent detachment — this can be done as an outpatient.

3 Those RDs that present with the macula on, i.e. central vision is good, have a good chance of retaining this vision postoperatively. If the macula is off, i.e. central vision is affected, than the visual prognosis is less predictable.

Retinal vein occlusion (CRVO and BRVO)

Typical presentation

As its name suggests this is a blockage of a retinal vein — if it is the central retinal vein it is a central retinal vein occlusion (CRVO), if it is one of its feeder veins it is a branch retinal vein occlusion (BRVO). Unlike central retinal artery occlusion, it is not an acute catastrophic event but takes some time for the vein to become critically narrowed. However once this critical rise in venous back pressure occurs the retina becomes ischaemic and the vision drops rapidly. Visual acuity can be very variable — if it is a complete CRVO the vision can be PL or HMS, whilst if it is a peripheral BRVO the vision may be unaltered.

Examination of the fundus reveals scattered "flame-shaped" retinal haemorrhages and sometimes cotton-wool spots. In CRVO these are maximal around the optic disc but should also be present further out in the retina. Haemorrhage around the disc itself suggests AION rather than vein occlusion. In BRVO the haemorrhage is only around the affected vein.

Principles of treatment

1 Patients with vein occlusions need referral to an ophthalmologist — usually within 48 hours.
2 Most patients have an underlying cause and this may require medical investigation.

How and what to do

1 Take a history bearing in mind the possible underlying causes for a vein occlusion — see below for these.

2 Examination must include visual acuity, check for an RAPD and dilate the pupils for fundoscopy. Look for flame-shaped haemorrhages and/or cotton-wool spots on the retina. The optic disc may be swollen, the main differential diagnosis for this is anterior ischaemic optic neuropathy. However the latter only has haemorrhages and cotton-wool spots (CWS) around the disc, while CRVO has them all over the fundus.

3 Patients with CRVO or BRVO need referral to an ophthalmologist for close follow-up and/or treatment. Because they produce retinal ischaemia new vessels can develop on the retina and trabecular meshwork causing vitreous haemorrhage and neovascular glaucoma. This latter process classically occurs 3 months after the occlusion (so-called 90-day glaucoma) and produces a particularly aggressive form of glaucoma that is difficult to treat and can be exquisitely painful.

4 Early referral to an ophthalmologist allows early detection of ischaemia and treatment with laser (pan-retinal photocoagulation as in diabetic retinopathy). Ischaemia is indicated by poor vision ($\sim$ HMS), an RAPD, large numbers of cotton-wool spots and large areas of ischaemia present on fluorescein angiography.

5 The majority of patients with CRVO or BRVO have an obvious cause:
   - systemic hypertension (commonest cause)
   - cardiovascular disease
   - cerebrovascular disease
   - hyperlipidaemias
   - diabetes.

Thus all patients must have their blood pressure, BM and urine checked as a minimum. If the patient is fit and well or is under 50 years of age they may benefit from a cardiology assessment. Occasionally hyperviscosity or clotting abnormalities are picked up in this way, e.g. lymphomas, leukaemias or macroglobulinaemias.

6 Prior to ophthalmic referral check the patient's blood pressure and urine (for glucose) and let the ophthalmologist know the results. If the blood pressure is greatly elevated in the presence of a unilateral or bilateral vein occlusion the patient needs referral to the on-call medical team before being referred on to the ophthalmologists.

7 Temporal arteritis does not present with venous occlusions and therefore an urgent ESR is not required.

8 It is not uncommon for patients who have had a unilateral vein occlusion for some time to present, having only noticed the decrease in vision after closing their good eye. Despite this apparent delay these patients also need immediate referral to exclude/confirm the diagnosis and look for signs of neovascularisation.

Vitreous haemorrhage

Typical presentation

Bleeding into the vitreous gel tends to occur as a sudden event, with patients noting a storm of red floaters. Depending on the amount of haemorrhage, vision can vary from near normal to hand movements. Examination reveals a reduced red reflex and usually fundal details cannot be seen. There are various causes of vitreous haemorrhage but these can be masked by the blood.

Principles of treatment

1 The most important question to answer is — what has caused the vitreous haemorrhage? The haemorrhage itself is not important as most will clear spontaneously, but the underlying cause may require urgent treatment.
2 The commonest causes of vitreous haemorrhage are:
   - bleeding new vessels from diabetic retinopathy
   - retinal detachment
   - bleeding new vessels from a central or branch retinal vein occlusion
   - posterior vitreous detachment.
   The history and examination are aimed at identifying this underlying cause.

How and what to do

1 Take a full history. Is the patient diabetic or hypertensive (vein occlusions)? Have they had this before and what was the cause. Have they had any systemic symptoms of diabetes? Are they on aspirin or warfarin?
2 Check the visual acuity in both eyes.

3 Check for an afferent pupillary defect. This is important as it indicates either ischaemic retina (i.e. diabetic retinopathy or vein occlusion) or a significant retinal detachment.

4 Dilate the pupils with tropicamide 1% or cyclopentolate 1%. Dilate both eyes as the fellow eye may well give clues to the underlying cause of the haemorrhage.

5 When dilated compare the two red reflexes. Attempt to see the fundus of the affected eye — it is often not possible and so gradually turn the ophthalmoscope dial to increasing plus (i.e. the red numbers) as it is sometimes possible to see large clumps of haemorrhage.

6 Full ophthalmic assessment is necessary so the patient needs referral within 24 hours. If the ophthalmologist cannot get a fundal view, ultrasound scanning of the eye is used to exclude a retinal detachment.

7 Prior to referral, check the patient's urine for glucose and check the BP. If the patient is on warfarin, check the INR.

8 Treatment depends on the cause. If the retina is detached the patient will undergo a vitrectomy (surgical removal of the vitreous) and RD repair. If the cause is benign, e.g. a PVD, time is given for the haemorrhage to clear by itself.

Decreased vision with pain

Acute closed angle glaucoma (ACAG)

Typical presentation

Acute closed angle glaucoma is a relatively sudden blockage of the trabecular meshwork (the drainage area for aqueous)that results in a rapid rise in IOP. It is this sudden rise in pressure that is responsible for the classic symptoms of ACAG — ocular pain, decreased vision, nausea, and vomiting. Examination reveals an injected eye with a marked decrease in vision. On gentle palpation, the eye feels hard and direct inspection usually shows a hazy ("steamy") cornea. The pupil is fixed in a mid-dilated position with no retinal view possible.

Atypical presentations can occur with abdominal pain, nausea and vomiting being the predominant symptoms and the presence of a red eye being overlooked by both patient and practitioner.

Although of apparently sudden onset, early warning symptoms can often occur for weeks or months prior to the full attack. These symptoms are in fact rises and falls in pressure typically occurring in the evening (when the pupil is relatively dilated). They cause ocular pain and the pressure forces fluid into the cornea causing what patients describe as "haloes" or "rainbows" around lights.

Principles of treatment

1 Both ACAG and its warning symptoms are ophthalmic emergencies and require immediate referral to eye casualty.
2 Do not dilate the pupil in order to get a look at the optic disc. This will exacerbate the angle closure — and the disc will not actually show any changes in the acute phase.
3 Treatment of ACAG involves immediate medical reduction of IOP and this should be done by an ophthalmologist. Definitive treatment after normalising the IOP is undertaken by punching a hole in the iris with a laser (peripheral iridectomy (Figure 2.12, page 62)).

What to do

1 Although most non-ophthalmologists will never see a patient with ACAG, if the presentation is typical, the diagnosis is usually self-evident.
2 The patient may well be in some distress when you see them. If nausea and vomiting are a problem give IM prochlorperazine 12.5 mg or IM metaclopramide 10 mg stat.
3 Take as much history as possible, especially asking about premonitory symptoms. Check the visual acuity, cornea and pupil — these quickly confirm the diagnosis.
4 Refer the patient by telephone and give details of past medical history and drug history. Most patients are admitted for treatment, so contact appropriate friends or family so that they can make arrangements.
5 For patients who have not had an acute attack but have the prodromal symptoms, discuss immediately with an ophthalmologist. Examination of these patients is often normal. **Do not** dilate the pupil to view the disc as this is likely to precipitate an acute attack.

6 ACAG can present in different guises, beware the confused, post-operative (any type of surgery involving a GA) or the patient with an acute abdomen and a red eye.

Optic neuritis (retrobulbar neuritis)

Typical presentation

Although the term optic neuritis is actually a non-specific term, it is used clinically to mean a self-limiting inflammation of the optic nerve. Patients, typically young females, complain of progressive reduction in vision over a few days associated with pain on eye movements. Improvement is spontaneous within 2 weeks of onset and often returns to normal within 3 months. Fifty per cent of patients go on to have a second episode — this is strongly suggestive of demyelinating disease.

Principles of treatment

1 Optic neuritis must be differentiated from other optic neuropathies.
2 All patients with a first attack of optic neuritis need to see an ophthalmologist to confirm or exclude the diagnosis.
3 Patients who have a second attack or other neurological problems need to see a neurologist to confirm or exclude demyelinating disease.

How and what to do

1 A first attack of optic neuritis can often be diagnosed from the history alone:
   - A first episode is rare after the age of 45 and even with typical features should only be diagnosed with caution.
   - Pain with eye movements and decreased vision in one eye is highly suggestive of optic neuritis.
   - The patient may complain of colours appearing to be "washed out".
   - If the symptoms get worse in heat (often a bath or a shower),

this is called Uthoff's phenomena and is typical of demyelinating disease.

2 Ask about other odd neurological symptoms that may have come and gone, such as paraesthesia, dizziness, shooting neck pains or limb weakness.

3 Visual acuity testing is vital:

- Visual acuity loss is very variable, ranging from 6/6 to NPL.
- Colour vision testing is important as it is almost always reduced (testing formally with Ishihara plates or even subjectively holding up a red target, see page 31) compared to the fellow eye.
- Reduced acuity and colour vision are not specific abnormalities found in optic neuritis but are indicative of any optic neuropathy (although not of papilloedema) and findings must be taken in the context of the history.

4 Patients with unilateral optic neuritis will have an afferent pupillary defect — this remains after the inflammation has settled but will disappear if the other eye becomes involved.

5 Patients with a first attack of optic neuritis need to be seen by an ophthalmologist to confirm the diagnosis. It is a matter for individual judgement if the association with multiple sclerosis is mentioned at this first presentation.

6 Patients with a second attack or other neurological symptoms should be referred to a neurologist. The role of MRI, steroids and beta-interferon varies between practitioners and areas. Oral steroids are now contraindicated in optic neuritis.

7 Although the differential diagnosis of optic neuropathies is long, the features of optic neuritis are usually fairly obvious:

- Take care in the patient over 50 with a first presentation — always do an urgent ESR in these patients before referring to eye casualty.
- Improvement in visual acuity should **begin** within 2 weeks of commencement. If this does not occur, further investigation is indicated.
- One condition that can mimic optic neuritis almost exactly is sphenoidal sinusitis — this can cause sudden visual loss, APD, decreased colour vision **and** pain with eye movements. It is tragic to miss it, as early sphenoidal sinus drainage can cure the optic neuropathy.
- Consider urgent CT scanning of the orbit and sinuses if the patient has a history of sinus disease or if the lids are puffy and tender.

Temporal arteritis

Typical presentation

Temporal arteritis (giant cell or cranial arteritis) is an inflammatory process affecting the medium sized arteries of the head and neck. It is closely associated with polymyalgia rheumatica and like PMR almost never occurs in patients under the age of 50.

Temporal arteritis classically presents with unilateral headache, tender scalp, anorexia, malaise, pyrexia and pain when chewing. Because it is an arteritic process symptoms and signs are related to blockage of small and medium sized blood vessels — in the eye this can manifest as sudden painless loss of vision (central retinal artery occlusion or anterior ischaemic optic neuropathy) or double vision (occlusion of vessels supplying the extraocular muscles).

Principles of treatment

1 Temporal arteritis is detected by having a high index of clinical suspicion.
2 If the patient has typical signs and symptoms of temporal arteritis they must be treated **immediately** — the ESR is important but produces a significant number of false positives and negatives.
3 Any patient who has sudden loss of vision or sudden onset of double vision should be questioned for the signs and symptoms of temporal arteritis and have an urgent ESR performed.
4 Temporal arteritis can blind the patient within hours, therefore once detected needs treatment immediately.
5 Treatment is with high-dose steroids and these are tailed off over a prolonged period. While temporal arteritis should not be missed, long-term steroids have their own problems and should only be used with justification.

How and what to do

1 The symptoms of temporal arteritis should be familiar to those dealing with eye patients — they are discussed on page 17, Section 1. The ideal situation is to make the diagnosis before the eye complications develop so that they can be prevented.

Unfortunately this does not always happen and the first presentation is with sudden loss of vision and, retrospectively, the symptoms can be seen to be have been present for some time.

2 If symptoms suggest temporal arteritis the patient needs a full systemic examination:
   - Often the patient actually looks unwell.
   - The patient seems lethargic and depressed.
   - There may be a slight pyrexia.
   - Sometimes the patient's clothes look too big because of the weight they have lost.
   - The affected temple(s) can be so tender to touch that the patient puts his/her hand up to stop you touching them.
   - The artery feels thick underneath the fingers and no pulse is detected — although even in definite temporal arteritis, the artery can feel completely normal.
   - The signs of AION and CRAO (temporal arteritis does not cause CRVO) are discussed in the appropriate topic, as are those of sudden onset of diplopia.
   - It is extremely important to look for temporal arteritis in **all** these patients — although, of course, the vast majority will not have it.

3 The ESR is often used in isolation to make or exclude the diagnosis of temporal arteritis. Unfortunately it is nowhere near sensitive or specific enough for this. The ESR can be well within the normal range (see page 70) and the patient has definite temporal arteritis, or it can be very high in patients with no signs or symptoms of the disease. The ESR should be considered in the context of signs and symptoms, the only exception to this would be if the patient had an acute CRAO or AION and a very high ESR and this will be discussed below.

4 Many practitioners feel that temporal artery biopsy (TAB) should be performed in all patients with temporal arteritis. The rationale is that the patient is going to be on long-term steroids and the risk of side effects makes a positive diagnosis important. TAB is usually of little use after a week's treatment with steroids.

5 When the diagnosis of temporal arteritis is suspected, treatment must begin immediately with IV methyl prednisolone 500 mg–1 g (given slowly over 15 min — check with data sheet if you are unsure) or IV hydrocortisone 200–300 mg (depending on the patient's size). Give 60–80 mg of oral prednisolone at the same time.

6 Once the steroids have been given the patient needs immediate referral. If the patient has no ocular symptoms refer by telephone

to a rheumatologist or the on-call physician. If there are ocular symptoms refer to eye casualty.

7 Because of the high-dose steroids, it is vital to know the patient's past medical history, e.g. diabetes, hypertension or tuberculosis. Baseline FBC, blood sugar, chest X-ray and blood pressure are taken as soon after admission as possible. Sugar and BP need close monitoring. Urinalysis should be undertaken and, if necessary, an MSU to rule out a UTI.

8 Treatment for temporal arteritis is likely to be long term — the vast majority of patient's disease continues for more than 2 years. Steroid dose is reduced slowly and the patient's symptoms and ESR titrated against the dose. Patients often have a remarkably fast improvement in their symptoms but it takes longer for the ESR to drop.

Lid, lash and lacrimal problems

Acute dacrocystitis

Typical presentation

This is an acute infection of the lacrimal sac. Patients present with pain, redness and tenderness over the area of the lacrimal sac (Figure 3.1). Occasionally patients can be systemically unwell and pyrexial. Most patients when questioned will give a long

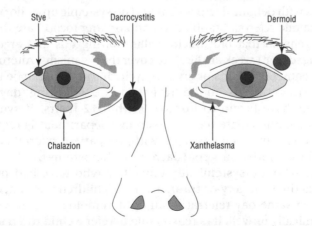

Figure 3.1 Composite diagram of location of various lid lumps and lesions.

history of nasolacrimal duct obstruction, i.e. a watering and occasionally discharging eye for months or years.

Principles of treatment

1 Treatment of the infection with appropriate antibiotics.
2 Acute dacrocystitis indicates that the lacrimal drainage system is blocked. When the infection has settled, surgery will be required to bypass this blockage.
3 If the redness and tenderness are more widespread or the patient is unwell, think of the possibility of a preseptal or orbital cellulitis.

How and what to do

1 Exclude an associated orbital cellulitis (see page 93), i.e. is there lid cellulitis, proptosis, restriction of eye movements, a reduction in visual acuity or an APD?
2 Take the patient's temperature.
3 Examine the inflamed area and apply firm but gentle pressure over the sac to see if any discharge is obtained from the lacrimal punctum. Take a microbiology (bacterial only) swab of any expressed discharge.
4 Do not try to irrigate the lacrimal system or incise the lacrimal sac when it is acutely inflamed — if the infection is "pointing" it is soon going to rupture onto the skin anyway.
5 Adults with definite dacrocystitis and no systemic upset do not need ophthalmic referral. Staphlococci and/or streptococci are the usual pathogens so that oral flucloxacillin 500 mg qds and amoxicillin 500 mg tds for 1 week are likely to cover the organisms. Alternatively, Augmentin 625 mg tds or erythromycin 500 mg qds can be used.
6 The patient needs to be reviewed the following day, most patients have begun to improve within 12 hours. If symptoms are worse immediate referral to an eye department is required.
7 Once this acute attack is dealt with, outpatient referral is necessary for definitive surgery (dacrocystorhinostomy).
8 Adults who are systemically unwell or who have had previous nasolacrimal surgery or trauma and all children with dacrocystitis need same-day referral to an ophthalmologist. If the child is systemically unwell, it is reasonable to refer a child to a paediatrician initially.

Common lid lesions

Some of these are illustrated in Figure 3.1.

Chalazion (old name internal hordoleum)

- This represents a blocked meibomian gland and is therefore found about 0.5 cm from the eyelid margin.
- Chalazia initially present as small, red, tender lumps but this inflammation (which is directed toward the lipid in the gland) slowly subsides over some weeks.
- Often a small, hard lump remains and can remain for months — although all tend to disappear eventually.
- They can become secondarily infected, when they increase in size and are surrounded by an area of cellulitis.

Treatment

- In the initial inflamed stage, warm compresses for 5–10 minutes three times a day may help. A warm face flannel is pressed over the lump and massaged upwards.
- Alternatively, prepacked face napkins as used in some Chinese restaurants (they can be bought in Chinese supermarkets) can be used.
- Antibiotic ointments or drops are ineffective for chalazia.
- If the lump persists for more than 6 months or is particularly troublesome, refer the patient for incisions and curettage.
- If there are signs of secondary infection/cellulitis treat with oral antibiotics, e.g. Tabs flucloxacillin 500 mg qds for 1 week.
- Chalazia are almost always associated with blepharitis and therefore this needs to be treated appropriately — this is described under "Blepharitis" (see page 118).

Stye (external hordoleum)

- This is an infected eyelash follicle and therefore is found at the lash margin (Figure 3.1).
- It has a short time-course and resolves spontaneously within a week.

- If a patient does present with one, use epilation forceps to remove the involved lash — this will hasten resolution.
- Styes do not need topical or systemic antibiotics (unless there is an obvious cellulitis).

Basal and squamous cell carcinomas

- Eyelids are on sun-exposed areas of skin and are prone to basal cell carcinomas and squamous cell carcinomas.
- Skin thickening, inflammation, ulceration, bleeding, telangiectasia and destruction of the local architecture should alert you to the possibility of malignancy.
- Suspicious lesions need referral to an ophthalmologist because of the peculiar anatomy of the eyelids.

Molluscum contagiosum

- These present usually as multiple tiny papules with umbilicated centres.
- When they arise near the lid margin they can shed virus into the conjunctiva causing a chronic conjunctivitis.
- They are self-limiting but if cosmetically embarrassing or causing conjunctivitis they can be removed.

Cyst of Moll and cyst of Zeiss

- These are small apocrine and sebaceous cysts found at the lash margin.
- They only need removal if the patient feels them to be unsightly.

Xanthelasma

- These are yellow plaques usually on the medial aspects of the lids (Figure 3.1).
- They consist of subcutaneous intracellular lipid deposits.
- They are associated with raised lipids and diabetes. A lipid profile and blood sugar are indicated, although most will be normal.

- If they are unsightly refer to an ophthalmologist or plastic surgeon for removal.

Dermoid

- Dermoid cysts are firm lesions usually found at the outer side of the eyebrow (Figure 3.1).
- They consist of epithelium and keratin but are deep to the skin.
- They are mobile but are usually tethered to the underlying bone.
- They are present at birth and grow with the child.
- Although benign they can rupture with resulting inflammation.
- Refer to an ophthalmologist any child with a possible dermoid.

Strawberry naevus

- These capillary haemangiomas can occur on the upper lid.
- They can cause amblyopia if large and are often associated with astigmatism.
- All need referral from birth for treatment and/or follow-up.

Ectropion and entropion

Typical presentation

Patients who have in-turning of their lower eyelid (entropion) have symptoms related to their lashes rubbing on the cornea and conjunctiva, i.e. a foreign body sensation, redness and discharge.

Patients with turning out of their lower lid (ectropion) have symptoms related to the pooling of tears by the lid and they get watering and recurrent discharge.

Principles of treatment

1 Think of the possible underlying cause although most are involutional (age related). Other causes include trauma, chemical injury, and traction on the lids, e.g. from lid lesions.
2 Definitive treatment is operative, does the patient want this?

3 Entropion abrades the cornea, therefore there is an increased risk of corneal infection.

How and what to do

1 **Take a history.** How long has the problem been present? Has there been any trauma? Chemical burn? Previous surgery? Any previous treatment?

2 **Examine the lids.** Is there a local cause for the problem, e.g. a lid lump or scarring? Is the lid turned outwards (ectropion) or inwards (entropion)? How healthy does the conjunctiva look — is it red and inflamed suggesting chronic exposure? Are the lashes touching the cornea?

3 Check corneal staining by instilling 2% fluoroscein. If there is staining the cornea needs to be protected and the patient referred.

4 Treatment for **entropion:**
   - If there is corneal staining protect the cornea with lubricating ointment, e.g. Occ. Simplex or Lacri-Lube qds. Drops do not offer prolonged protection. If the patient gets a conjunctivitis, treat with Occ. chloramphenicol qds for a week.
   - As a temporary measure tape the lid away from the globe (Figure 3.2). Teach a relative or friend of the patient to do this. Using surgical tape cut pieces to about 10 cm, apply gentle traction on the lid skin so that the lid is everted to a

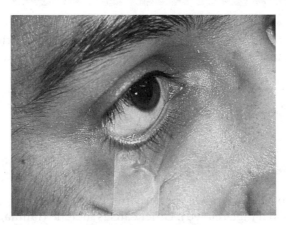

Figure 3.2 Taping the lower lid away from the globe as a temporary measure for correction of entropion.

normal position; tape the lid in this position. Tell the patient (or relative) to re-tape if it becomes loose.
 – Refer the patient and inform the patient to return immediately if symptoms worsen.
5 Treatment for **ectropion**:
 – If there is corneal staining treat with lubricating ointment as described above.
 – Use antibiotic ointment, e.g. Occ. chloramphenicol tds, if the conjunctiva is inflamed.
 – Refer the patient and inform him/her to return immediately if symptoms worsen.

Lash epilation

• Occasionally patients present with one or two in-turned lashes — this may be a one-off or a chronic problem.
• Examine the lids with a good light or slit-lamp if you have one and identify the offending lashes.
• They should be removed with epilation forceps — which are the same as those that can be bought from a high street chemist.
• Grab the base of the lash with the forceps and pull it vertically up or down depending which lid.
• If the lashes are too small and flexible to be gripped by the forceps then it is unlikely that they are causing any symptoms and do not need removal.
• Check for corneal staining with 2% fluorescein. If present give Occ. or g. chloramphenicol tds for 3 days, if there is no staining antibiotics are not needed.
• If there are a large number of lashes or the patient is having frequent problems refer the patient for consideration of lash root destruction with electrolysis or cryotherapy.

Facial (VIIth nerve) palsy

Typical presentation

Patients present with weakness affecting one side of the face, inability to shut the eye, inability to show facial expressions or drooling from the side of the mouth. The onset may be acute and unexpected or associated with recent intracranial surgery.

The term "Bell's palsy" is often incorrectly used to describe any facial palsy, it should in fact be reserved for the idiopathic type, i.e. it is a diagnosis of exclusion.

Principles of treatment

1 Is there a sinister underlying cause for the facial palsy? It is important to differentiate between central or peripheral causes of VIIth nerve palsy and to be aware of associated causes that may be life threatening.
2 The main ocular morbidity comes from incomplete eyelid closure. The cornea needs normal lid and tear function to remain healthy and if this environment is altered there is a significant risk of permanent corneal scarring. The cornea needs to be protected until the paralysis recovers.

How and what to do

General examination

1 The purpose of a full history and examination is to look for signs and symptoms that suggest that further neurological investigation is required. The purpose of the eye examination is to assess the amount of corneal exposure.
2 Potentially suspicious symptoms include:
   – persistent pain
   – facial paraesthesia
   – facial anaesthesia
   – any additional neurological symptoms
   – headache, nausea or vomiting (meningism)
   – skin rashes (think of lyme disease)
   – cough and night sweats (sarcoidosis)
   – gradual onset of the pareses and lack of improvement after 1 month.
   – loss of taste and hyperacusis are not suspicious in themselves as they often accompany Bell's palsy.
3 Complete examination of the cranial nerves, especially concentrating on the Vth and VIIth cranial nerves, is mandatory

and any associated cranial nerve palsies are suspicious. It is often stated that corneal sensation (Vth nerve) should be normal, in fact corneal exposure often significantly reduces corneal sensation and can be misleading. Vth nerve function is more reliably tested by touching the nasal mucosa with cotton wool.

4 It is extremely important to determine whether the cause of the facial palsy is central or peripheral. This is achieved by asking the patient to wrinkle his/her forehead, if the lesion is central (i.e. in the brain), wrinkling is possible (there is crossing of central fibres and upper facial musculature is bilaterally supplied). If the patient cannot wrinkle the brow the palsy has a peripheral nerve cause (weakness affecting all facial musculature). This incomplete facial involvement is a suspicious sign.

5 Examine the ear, external auditory meatus, head and neck for zoster-like vesicles. Ramsey–Hunt syndrome is a herpes zoster infection of the outer ear that can cause a facial weakness. Treatment is with either aciclovir 800 mg 5 times a day for a week or famciclovir 250 mg tds for 1 week.

6 Palpate the parotid gland for masses.

7 Check for eyelid synkinesis, i.e. is there any sign of aberrant regeneration of nerve fibres? This is seen either as contraction of the corner of the mouth with attempted eyelid closure or tearing when chewing (crocodile tears) and is an indication of chronicity.

8 If there are no suspicious features and the eye appears adequately protected referral is not necessary. If you are suspicious of a serious underlying cause refer urgently to a neurologist. If the ocular surface is compromised (see below) refer to an ophthalmologist the same day.

9 Most Bell's palsies are spontaneously improved after a month. Oral steroids do not seem to have an effect on the rapidity of improvement and may mask underlying pathology.

Ocular examination

1 Is the cornea at risk of damage from exposure? Check:
   - Visual acuity.
   - Orbicularis strength — ask the patient to shut his/her eyes and determine how difficult it is for you to force open the lids.
   - Look for ectropion — turning out of lower lid can indicate the eye may be drying quickly.
   - Bell's phenomenon — while keeping the lids open, ask the patient to shut his/her eyes, how much does the eye rotate

upwards (normally it should almost disappear)? If there is a poor Bell's phenomenon then the cornea is at much greater risk of damage.
  – Check for exposure keratopathy by instilling 2% fluoroscein and checking for corneal staining with a blue light. Exposure results in scattered loss of epithelial cells so that a spotty pattern of flourescein is seen.
2 If the cornea appears healthy and the lids can be forcibly closed by the patient, prophylactic measures are needed:
  – Use lubricating ointment, e.g. Occ. simplex or Lacri-Lube qds.
  – Instruct the patient to tape the lid shut at night after adding ointment.
  – Warn the patient that the ointment can smear the vision for some time — especially as the poor lid function means that the ointment is washed away more slowly (which is of course the reason for using it).
  – Occ. chloramphenicol qds can be used if there is a discharge or if hygiene is a problem.
3 If there are any signs of corneal exposure or if lid function is very poor, refer to an ophthalmologist immediately.
4 If lid function does not improve over time, lid surgery may be undertaken to improve coverage (tarsorraphy).

Herpes zoster (shingles)

Typical presentation

Herpes zoster ophthalmicus (HZO) is a reactivation of the herpes zoster virus (from a previous infection clinically manifested as chickenpox) in the first division of the trigeminal ganglion, i.e. on the head, forehead, upper lid, eye and the nose down to its tip. It usually only affects one division and it is therefore unilateral — stopping at the centre of the forehead and nose. Patients are usually over 60, the initial symptom is periocular pain, which is followed 24–48 hours later by a vesicular skin rash. The vesicles crust over in a few days although the skin lesions can persist for some weeks.

Around 50% of patients with HZO get ocular complications ranging from mild and self-limiting to sight threatening. The diagnosis is obvious once the typical vesicular skin rash of herpes zoster (localised to a dermatome and does not cross the midline) becomes apparent. Pain may be a prominent feature, the lids are swollen, and the patient may or may not have a red eye.

Principles of treatment

1 Early recognition of the disease is important both to rule out other disease (e.g. temporal arteritis or lid cellulitis) and to begin treatment.
2 Early recognition of eye involvement is also important and needs referral.
3 General supportive measures, especially in the very elderly.
4 Adequate pain relief during the course of the disease.
5 Remember that HZO can be the presenting feature of an immuno-compromised patient. The vast majority of patients with HZO are not immunocompromised but the likelihood increases if more than one dermatome is involved.

How and what to do

1 Because the first symptom of HZO is often temporal/periorbital pain it may be mistaken in the early stages for temporal arteritis. Once the characteristic rash develops the diagnosis becomes obvious.
2 Once the rash develops start the patient on either aciclovir 800 mg 5 times a day for 1 week or valaciclovir 1 g tds for 1 week. They reduce the incidence of ocular side effects and may reduce the incidence of post herpetic neuralgia. They are only effective during the early stages of the disease and a useful guide is only prescribe them if the patient still has vesicles. Patients should be advised to keep up a good fluid intake with these treatments.
3 The patients, often elderly, may feel quite unwell during the first week and general support is needed. Bed rest may help and fluids are very important. If a frail patient lives alone it may be worth considering admitting them to hospital.
4 Adequate analgesia is important — both to make the patient more comfortable during the acute stages and because there is evidence that it reduces the risk of postherpetic neuralgia.
5 If the patient has no ocular symptoms during the course of the disease then they do not need an ophthalmic opinion. However, the range of eye complications — from keratoconjunctivitis,

uveitis, scleritis to retinitis, optic neuritis and cranial nerve palsies — is so great that any eye symptoms (as opposed to lid symptoms) need immediate referral.

6 If the eyelids become very swollen they can completely close the eye — if this prevents examination of the eye, refer to an ophthalmologist.

7 It is not unusual for oedema from the affected skin to track to the other side of the face (especially if the patient has been lying on this side). Whilst this is alarming it is not sinister and will resolve quickly, especially if the patient sits up.

8 Hutchinson's sign in HZO — if the area of skin supplied by the nasociliary nerve is affected by the rash then the incidence of ocular involvement is much higher than if it were not. This area of skin is the side and tip of the nose. Around 80% of those with the sign have ocular involvement and if present you should have a high index of suspicion.

9 Postherpetic neuralgia is pain in the same dermatome as the rash that persists after the active disease, usually for 1–2 years but sometimes for much longer. Studies are contradictory as to whether early, oral aciclovir reduces its incidence — oral steroids do not seem to have an effect. Once established many different treatments have been tried but most are disappointing — early referral to a pain specialist may be beneficial.

10 The skin lesions of HZO do not necessarily need specific treatment, but should be kept clean. If particularly severe or troublesome to the patient, aciclovir 5% (the eye ointment is 3%) applied to the lesions 5 times a day for 1 week may help.

11 The skin lesions can become secondarily bacterially infected — manifested by a marked increase in pain and local redness. It can be treated with oral flucloxacillin 500 mg qds or erythromycin 500 mg qds.

12 HZO is common in immunocompromised patients but it is relatively rare for immune deficiency to present in this way. This is more likely (but still uncommon) if more than one dermatome is involved or if the patient is a child. If this situation arises or there are other suspicious features of immunocompromise, refer immediately to an infectious diseases physician.

13 It is worth remembering that the HZO vesicles contain live virus and it is therefore possible for someone not previously exposed to the virus to catch chickenpox from someone with shingles (it is of course not possible for them to "catch" shingles). Infectivity ends when the last vesicle has gone.

Lid twitching

Patients may be very troubled by involuntary twitching, blinking and intermittent closure of their eyelids.

Eyelid myokymia

- This is a very common occurrence and is a small area of fasciculation of the orbicularis muscle.
- Patients present having noticed an irritating twitch around one eye. It has no sinister underlying cause and resolves spontaneously.
- It appears to be related to tiredness — some patients find excess caffeine or nicotine can trigger it.
- Facial myokymia (which is much more widespread on the face) is completely different and can have an underlying sinister cause.
- There is no specific treatment. Reassurance is important and it is probably helpful to suggest rest and reducing caffeine intake.

Essential blepharospasm

- Blepharospasm is an involuntary, persistent, and forcible contraction of the entire orbicularis resulting in firm closure of the eyelids.
- Essential (or primary) blepharospasm is not secondary to ocular disease (although it can be worsened by ocular factors such as blepharitis) but is a disease of unknown aetiology.
- It needs to be separated from hemifacial spasm and referral to a neurologist is required.
- It often responds well to botulinum toxin injections but they have to be repeated.

Preseptal and orbital cellulitis

Typical presentation

Differentiating between preseptal and orbital cellulitis is extremely important. The orbital septum is a sheet of connective tissue that is attached to the rim of the orbit and separates the lids from the orbit and its contents. Infection behind the septum, i.e. within the orbit, is potentially life threatening as there is a direct route to the brain via the cavernous sinus. Lid infections are not life threatening because the orbital septum prevents extension of infection — thus they are called preseptal cellulitis. Having said that, untreated preseptal cellulitis can eventually lead to orbital cellulitis, especially in children.

Preseptal cellulitis presents as a unilateral swollen, red and very tender lid — the presence of pain/tenderness is important as it differentiates it from an allergic phenomena (see page 12). Adults are systemically well and apyrexial.

Orbital cellulitis presents in a similar manner with a unilateral, swollen, red and tender lid but there are important additional features, including proptosis and decreased vision. Additionally patients are systemically unwell with features ranging from anorexia and pyrexia to unconsciousness.

Principles of treatment

1 Preseptal cellulitis in adults is treated with oral antibiotics.
2 Preseptal cellulitis in children is treated with IV antibiotics.
3 Orbital cellulitis is an ophthalmic emergency in adults or children.
4 Orbital cellulitis is managed using a multidisciplinary approach.

How and what to do

1 **History and examination:**
   - The presence of severe lid infection, i.e. preseptal or orbital cellulitis is usually immediately apparent.
   - If it is a mild preseptal cellulitis the presence of pain will separate it from the superficially similar looking allergic lid disease.
   - Ask the patient (or parents) how long the symptoms have been present. How are they feeling in themselves? Hot? Thirsty? Drowsy?
   - These questions are vital for detecting possible extension of infection.
   - A history of sinus disease is important, as orbital cellulitis is most commonly caused by extension of infection from the ethmoid sinuses.
   - Observe the patient before carrying out any examination. Does the patient look ill?
   - Check the temperature, pulse and blood pressure.

- Check the visual acuity in both eyes, if the affected lids are so swollen that they are closed, gently prise the lids apart using gloves or a piece of gauze on each lid (it may be easier if an assistant does this).
- As the acuity is being checked, compare the two eyes. Is the affected globe protruded forward?
- Ask the patient to look up/down/left and right — limitation of any movements is strongly suggestive of orbital cellulitis.
- Examine for an RAPD — the presence of one is suggestive of optic nerve compression, i.e. orbital involvement of infection.
- If possible, check the colour vision in both eyes — if reduced in the affected eye this is another sign of optic nerve compression.
- Attempt to examine the optic nerve, but do not dilate the pupil (unless the infection is obviously preseptal) as this makes later assessment more difficult.

2 Sinus X-rays will not add to the diagnosis, if the patient has any signs of orbital cellulitis a CT scan of orbit and brain is required.

3 In essence, preseptal cellulitis is an infection of the lids and nothing else, so if there are **any** additional features, either ocular or systemic, it should be assumed that the patient has or is developing an orbital cellulitis.

4 **Management depends on the findings.**

Adults with preseptal cellulitis:
- These patients do not need referral under normal circumstances.
- Prescribe flucloxacillin 500 mg qds and amoxicillin 500 mg tds p.o. or erythromycin 500 mg qds p.o.
- Instruct the patient to return immediately if feeling unwell, their vision changes or their eye becomes more painful.
- Review at 24 hours when the patient should be more comfortable. Repeat the history and examination at this stage. If the patient is improving continue the antibiotics for 1 week.

Children with preseptal cellulitis:
- Because of the ease with which infection can pass through the orbital septum in children, they need admission for IV antibiotics.
- They can be referred to an ophthalmologist or a paediatrician first, but they need treatment and monitoring on a paediatric ward.

Orbital cellulitis:
- Patients with orbital cellulitis should be referred as an emergency to an ophthalmologist.
- ENT and/or neurosurgical opinions are often required, or paediatric if the patient is a child.

- Once admitted, IV antibiotics are begun prior to CT scanning.
- If an orbital abscess is present it is drained.
- Daily vision, colour vision and pupil responses are mandatory, looking for optic nerve compression.

Ptosis

Typical presentation

Ptosis means drooping of the eyelid. It may be congenital or acquired. It may be an isolated event (e.g. involutional ageing changes to the lid), caused purely by eye problems (e.g. contact lens wear), or it may be associated with an important underlying condition (e.g. Horner's syndrome). Patients usually present because it is cosmetically troubling or because it is interfering with their vision.

Principles of treatment

1 Rule out an underlying sinister cause for the ptosis.
2 Is the patient sufficiently troubled by the ptosis to want to undergo an operation to correct it?

How and what to do

1 Take a careful history.
   Features that are suggestive of serious underlying pathology:
   - Sudden onset (days or weeks).
   - Pain — ocular or headache.
   - If the pupil is dilated in the eye on the **same side** as a very marked ptosis, think of a IIIrd nerve palsy.
   - If the pupil is (apparently) dilated on the **opposite side** as a small ptosis, think of Horner's syndrome (it is in fact the pupil on the ptotic eye that is **constricted**).
   - If the patient has a marked diurnal variation in the degree of ptosis, i.e. no ptosis on first waking in the mornings but a severe ptosis by the evenings, think of myasthenia gravis.
   Features that tend to exclude serious underlying pathology:
   - Long history (years).
   - Family history of ptosis.

- No pupil involvement or squint.
- History of onset after accidental or surgical trauma.
- Bilateral.

2 If any suspicious features are present refer to a neurologist the same day.

3 If no suspicious features are found then further management depends on the patient.
- If the patient is a child, always refer them to an ophthalmologist — this is not necessarily for surgery but to monitor their visual development as ptosis can cause amblyopia.
- If the patient is an adult and feels the ptosis is cosmetically embarrassing or is obscuring their vision, it is necessary to warn him/her that surgery will be required. If the patient is prepared to undergo surgery, then refer routinely to an ophthalmologist.

4 Occasionally, in a patient with sight-interfering ptosis but who is not fit for surgery or who does not want it, special glasses can be made that have a "prop" attached that can mechanically lift the lid.

Thyroid eye disease (TED)

Typical presentation

Thyroid eye disease is an autoimmune process that can have a variety of different effects on the eye and orbit — from mild conjunctival irritation, to optic nerve compression, to severe limitation of extraocular muscle movements.

Eye symptoms may be the initial presentation of thyroid disease or may come on some time after the thyroid dysfunction has been diagnosed. Patients can present with a number of different symptoms, e.g. puffy lids, proptosis, decreased vision, double vision, or gritty eyes.

Principles of treatment

1 Any patient with recent onset of proptosis, diplopia, lid swelling or optic disc swelling needs to have their thyroid status checked.

2 Although commonest in those with hyperthyroidism (Grave's disease), TED can occur in hypothyroidism and in those who are biochemically euthyroid.

3 Patients with TED and their practitioners should be aware that TED is not a static disease, if patients notice that their visual acuity or colour vision is declining (optic nerve compression), or they have sudden onset or worsening of diplopia or that their eye is more gritty and sore (possible increased corneal exposure), they should be seen within 48 hours by an ophthalmologist.

4 It is important to recognise early optic nerve compression. It occurs more commonly in those with only minimal proptosis.

5 There is evidence that treatment with immunosuppression early in the course of TED can reduce the orbital involvement in the disease process.

How and what to do

Patients not known to have thyroid abnormalities who present with features of TED:

1 Why has the patient presented? Has the vision been affected? Are the eyes uncomfortable? If so are they worse in the mornings (poor lid closure)? Is there double vision?

2 Take a full systemic history especially looking for symptoms of thyroid disease. TED is commonest in hyperthyroidism but can occur in those who are hypothyroid or euthyroid.

3 Whatever the presenting symptoms a complete ophthalmic examination is necessary:
   - Check the visual acuity.
   - Check the colour vision — reduced colour vision can be the first sign of optic nerve compression.
   - Examine for proptosis — looking from above and behind the patient (see page 45).
   - Check the ocular movements (see page 37).
   - Confrontation field tests (see page 33).
   - Test for an APD — this can be a very subtle sign of optic nerve compression.
   - Instill 2% fluorescein and look for any areas of epithelial loss — these may indicate corneal exposure.

- Check the optic nerve for disc swelling with or without dilating the pupil.
4 To confirm the diagnosis blood will need to be taken for TFTs including TSH (and T_3/T_4 if possible) **and** for thyroid auto-antibodies.
5 If the TFTs are abnormal then refer to an endocrinologist.
6 Immediate ophthalmic referral is necessary if:
   - There are any signs of optic neuropathy, e.g. reduction or asymmetry in colour vision, an APD, optic disc swelling.
   - There are any signs of corneal exposure.
   - There is diplopia.
   - There are unexplained visual changes.
7 Irritation alone can be treated with g. hypromellose — this can be used as often as the patient finds necessary.
8 If there are signs or symptoms of exposure at night prescribe Occ. Simplex to be instilled very last thing at night. If this does not work, try taping the lids before sleep.
9 If cosmesis is a problem for the patient refer to an orbital/oculoplastic surgeon.

Patients known to have thyroid dysfunction

Some patients may not have TED until they have been dysthyroid for some years. Generally the principles of history and examination are the same as those described above. The most important thing is for the patient and practitioner to be aware of the symptoms that can herald sight-threatening sequelae. Warn the patient to attend immediately if:

1 They notice a sudden decline in vision.
2 Their eye becomes red and sore.
3 They notice that colours seem "washed-out".
4 They get double vision.

Patients known to have thyroid eye disease

Similarly, patients who are known to have TED and are under an ophthalmologist or endocrinologist can have changes in their symptoms. Once again, patients need to be aware that any changes in their vision must be reported immediately to a supervising doctor.

The watering eye (epiphora)

Typical presentation

There is a wide range of causes — both pathological and physiological — of watering. This section deals with one of the commonest causes — a blocked nasolacrimal duct (NLD). Watering eyes caused by malfunction of tear drainage is called epiphora. It tends to present in one of three situations: in babies during the first year of life, in the elderly, and in those who have suffered lid or midfacial trauma that has damaged the tear drainage apparatus. Because of stasis of tears in the nasolacrimal system, discharge can also be a major symptom.

Principles of treatment

1 Bear in mind that there are many other causes of a watering/sticky eye.
2 90% of babies with congenital NLD obstruction will have spontaneous resolution by their first birthday.
3 Elderly patients are often not troubled enough by their symptoms to justify surgery.
4 NLD blockage is a risk factor for infection of the lacrimal sac (dacrocystitis).

How and what to do

Epiphora in babies

1 Take a history:
  - Typically the eyes have watered from about 3 months of age (when tear production increases).
  - Discharge and stickiness are intermittent and often quickly settle with antibiotic drops.
  - Photophobia is **not** a symptom of NLD obstruction — it is often indicative of other pathologies, e.g. congenital glaucoma or a corneal foreign body.
1 Examine the eyes and lids:
  - The lashes may be crusty.
  - Tears may be seen coming from between the lids.

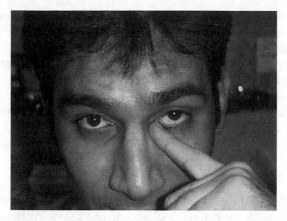

Figure 3.3 Pressing gently over the lacrimal sac when examining the watering eye.

- Press gently over the area of the lacrimal sac (Figure 3.3), this often causes regurgitation of discharge into the eye (this is not uncomfortable for the baby) and is a good sign of NLD obstruction.
- The conjunctivae should not be particularly injected but they may be slightly pink.
- The cornea should be bright and reflect the examining light.
- Check for the presence of the red reflex.
- Instill fluorescein 2%, check for corneal staining (should be absent with NLD obstruction). It is also useful to know that when the NLD is not obstructed all fluorescein should have drained away within 5 minutes — if there is still some around after this it is suggestive of obstruction.

3 **Management:**
  - 90% of NLD obstruction will settle spontaneously at 1 year.
  - It is important to explain this to the parents and to put their minds at rest.
  - They can clean the eye with some cool, boiled water when it becomes sticky — if it is very sticky a short course of topical antibiotics is helpful, e.g. Fucithalmic bd for 1 week.
  - It may also be helpful for parents to massage the lacrimal sac once or twice a day, this involves gently placing a finger on the sac area (see Figure 3.3) and running it up towards the eye. Although there is no evidence this may help clear the NLD obstruction.

- If the watering continues after a year, refer to an ophthalmologist for consideration of syringing and probing of the duct (this is done under a general anaesthetic).
- If the baby has an episode of dacrocystitis refer to an ophthalmologist immediately (see p. 81).
- The only symptoms of NLD obstruction are watering and discharge. If any other symptoms are present, have a low threshold for referral.

Epiphora in adults

1 Epiphora in adults occurs as a result of involutional changes in the NLD with eventual blockage of the tears. Although this is probably quite common, there is a reduction in tear production at around the same time and this may balance things out.
2 Examination is similar to the child's:
   - Look for discharge and press over the area of the sac.
   - There may be a lump over the sac area that is caused by a build up of mucus in the lacrimal sac (called a mucocoele) — this can be differentiated from dacrocystitis as it is not tender.
3 NLD obstruction in adults cannot be treated by probing the duct as it can in children and a new passage between the lacrimal sac and nasal mucosa needs to be formed (called a dacrocystorhinostomy). If elderly patients have ephiphora, it is worth asking them if it bothers them enough to have an operation before referring them.
4 Dacrocystitis is an indication for surgery as it is likely to be recurrent.
5 Massage of the sac does not work in adults.
6 Treat any associated conjunctivitis with topical antibiotics, e.g. g. chloramphenical qds for 1 week.

Ephiphora after lid or mid-facial trauma

1 This is a not uncommon situation and often occurs in young adults who are particularly troubled by it.
2 If the trauma has been recent it is worth waiting some months for it to settle spontaneously. If it does not, refer routinely to an ophthalmologist.
3 In the referral letter, give as many details of the trauma as you have.

Eye movement problems

The child with a squint

Typical presentation

A squint is the condition in which both eyes are not directed at the same object. The term strabismus has the same meaning. It is a relatively common condition of childhood and can be caused by a difference in refractive errors between the two eyes, poor vision in one eye, ocular muscle imbalance, or as part of a diverse range of syndromes.

Whilst adults whose eyes are not directed at the same object tend to present because they have double vision, children do not. This is because their brain suppresses the second image very quickly — something which adults cannot usually do. The typical presentation is when a parent or grandparent notices the child squinting or when there is a family history of squint.

Principles of treatment

1 Always believe the parents/grandparents or great aunts when they say they think the child has squinted, whatever your own findings are.
2 Always refer a child with a suspected squint to an orthoptist or ophthalmologist.
3 The vast majority of squints have no serious underlying cause but it is wise to be aware of the possibility when examining the child.

How and what to do

1 When taking the history ask how long the squint has been present. Does it come and go? Is there a family history of squint? Is the child well otherwise or has there been a recent change in health or behaviour?
2 Parents often get confused by the word squint — in an ophthalmic sense it does not mean screwing your eyes shut in bright light. Make sure at the start of the consultation that you and the patient are talking about the same thing.

3 It is very common for children under the age of 3 months to have an **intermittent** squint — it is only unusual if the squint is constant or if an intermittent squint persists after 3 months.

4 When examining the child:
   - Look and see how the child is behaving.
   - Try to check the vision one eye at a time (see Section 2 for a full description of visual assessment). If the child finds this upsetting do not force things — it is important that the child does not begin to associate having an eye examination with unpleasant experiences.
   - Shine a pen-torch light into the child's eyes and wait for the child to look at it — the two reflections should be in the same position on each cornea, if not there may be a squint present.
   - Move the pen-torch from side to side and up and down and get the child to follow it with their eyes, i.e. the child needs to keep the head still. If a pen-torch does not work use a toy for the child to follow.
   - Using the ophthalmoscope held at arm's length look for a red reflex — this is extremely important.

5 All children with squints need prompt (~4–6 weeks) orthoptic and ophthalmic referral. Referrals need not be urgent unless certain features are present:
   - If there is no red reflex.
   - If you cannot get the eye to move into all positions of gaze this suggests an ocular muscle problem.
   - The child has other suspicious ocular or neurological problems.

6 Children are not patched to correct their squint but to improve vision in an amblyopic eye. Amblyopia is decreased visual acuity without any detectable organic disease of the eye and can be thought of as resulting from suppression of the squinting eye. It is patching of the **good** eye which can cause the suppression to be reversed.

Adults with squints

- Although it was said in the introduction to this topic that adults tend to present with double vision rather than with the squint itself, this is not always true.
- If the patient already has poor vision in the squinting eye they will not perceive double vision.

- Alternatively, if the patient has had a squint as a child he/she can get a secondary deviation as an adult — this again may not cause diplopia because that eye has been suppressed.
- Adults who have squints that they find cosmetically unacceptable can be referred to an ophthalmologist for treatment.

Double vision (diplopia)

Typical presentation

Double vision (diplopia) is the perception of seeing two objects when only one is present. It is invariably due to an ocular muscle imbalance (although the eye muscles themselves need not be abnormal) between the two eyes.

True diplopia is only perceived when both eyes are open. If the diplopia persists with one eye closed this is called monocular diplopia — this is really a misnomer as it is not possible to get two separate images with one eye. Monocular diplopia is really seeing an "edge" to objects usually caused by refractive errors or cataract, while in true diplopia the patient will see the object and a second image of it separate (horizontally or vertically) from the object.

Principles of treatment

1 Separate monocular diplopia from binocular.
2 All patients with true diplopia need same-day referral to an eye casualty.
3 Patients with monocular diplopia can be referred to their optometrist for review.

How and what to do

1 The typical history and examination of a patient with double vision is described on pages 8 and 37.
2 In essence if the patient fixes on a target and one eye is covered — if the diplopia disappears it is true binocular, if it remains then it is monocular. This should then be repeated for the other eye.

3 Sudden onset of binocular diplopia requires immediate ophthalmic referral. Before referring check:
   - blood pressure
   - urine for sugar
   - if possible do an urgent ESR.

   Systemic hypertension, diabetes and temporal arteritis are three of the commonest causes of acute palsies.
4 If the double vision is associated with a dilated pupil and ptosis in the same eye (i.e. an acute IIIrd nerve palsy) refer immediately to a neurosurgeon to rule out a posterior communicating artery aneurysm. Remember that if the ptosis is complete the double vision will disappear!
5 If the patient has a past history of diplopia of known cause, e.g. thyroid disease, myasthenia gravis, but symptoms are worse, contact the patient's ophthalmologist for advice.
6 For monocular diplopia the patient should be referred to their own optometrist for an up-to-date eye test.
7 Do not allow patients with recent onset of diplopia to drive — they should contact the DVLA for advice.

Painful red eye

Acute anterior uveitis (AAU)

Typical presentation

Acute anterior uveitis is an inflammatory process of the eye which can occur as an isolated event, secondary to other eye diseases or as part of a systemic disease. Uveitis itself is an inflammation of the uveal tract (iris, ciliary body, and choroid) and therefore can occur at any location in the eye — although the commonest site is anterior. Anterior uveitis most commonly occurs secondary to some other ocular pathology, e.g. herpetic keratitis, scleritis or postoperatively.

AAU presents as a painful red, photophobic eye and the patient has usually noticed a reduction in vision. It is usually unilateral but can be bilateral. Patients may complain of pain when reading — this is because reading causes the iris to constrict and the pain is the movement of the inflamed iris. Careful examination using the slit-lamp allows visualisation of inflammatory cells in the anterior chamber and the posterior cornea (called keratic precipitates).

Without the slit-lamp these inflammatory cells can only be seen if they form reasonably large clumps — if the inflammation is severe the inflammatory cells will collect at the base of the anterior chamber and form something that looks like a snow-drift called a hypopyon (see Figure 3.4, p. 110).

Principles of treatment

1 When the patient presents with typical signs and symptoms of AAU, they need same-day referral to an ophthalmologist.
2 When the patient presents with typical signs and symptoms of AAU but they have recently had intraocular surgery they need immediate referral to an ophthalmologist to rule out an early endophthalmitis.
3 If a patient has had a previous episode of AAU and feels as if they are beginning to have a recurrence they are usually correct.
4 Patients with isolated AAU but no systemic symptoms do not need blanket investigations to look for an underlying cause.

How and what to do

1 The important symptoms of AAU are:
   – photophobia
   – pain
   – reduced vision
   – pain when reading or doing close work.
2 Symptoms of AAU do **not** include discharge/stickiness, irritation, itch, nausea and vomiting.
3 Important signs of AAU:
   – Redness (especially the conjunctiva near to the cornea).
   – Discomfort when being examined with the slit-lamp or ophthalmoscope.
   – Reduced visual acuity — although this can be very variable.
   – Inflammatory cells may be seen on the cornea or anterior chamber (see above).
   – The inflammatory products can make the iris very "sticky" and can form attachments to the front of the lens (see Figure 2.8, p. 42) — these are called synaechiae.
   – They can make the pupil difficult to dilate, although when it does the synaechiae are often more obvious.

- Difficulty in pupil dilation can make the retina, or even the red reflex, difficult to see.
- A useful sign in diagnosing uveitis is that the patients feel much more comfortable after pupil dilation — this is because dilation stops the inflamed iris moving.

4 AAU needs to be treated by an ophthalmologist no matter how often the patient has had previous recurrences. Intensive topical steroids are required and therefore ophthalmic supervision is needed, the pupil is dilated with g. atropine 1% bd or g. cyclopentolate 1% tds to increase comfort and to try to break the synaechiae.

5 AAU is usually a self-limiting disease and settles within 6 weeks (if not it becomes chronic uveitis). The topical steroid is slowly tailed off during this period. The mydriatic is usually stopped before this. If atropine is used to dilate the pupil its effect can last for up to 2 weeks after stopping, whereas the effect of cyclopentolate has passed after 8 hours. Patients should be warned that these drops will cause their pupil to be very large, they will have difficulty reading from the dilated eye, and that they should not drive until the drops are stopped. G. atropine should not be used in children.

6 Although it has many systemic associations, most patients who have AAU do not have an underlying systemic association. Of those that do, the disease is usually known about when they present with a first episode of AAU. It is important to ask about skin, joint, gastrointestinal, back and genitourinary symptoms when the patient presents but investigation is only indicated if these symptoms are positive. Certain ocular features increase the likelihood of an underlying systemic cause, e.g. bilateral AAU or retinal/vitreous involvement. Some systemic associations of AAU:
- **Skin** e.g. psoriasis, Behçet's disease
- **Joint** e.g. ankylosing spondylitis, juvenile chronic arthritis
- **GI** e.g. ulcerative colitis, Crohn's disease
- **GU** e.g. Reiter's syndrome
- **Respiratory** e.g. sarcoidosis, TB.

7 AAU in children is much more likely to have a systemic cause — often one of the juvenile arthropathies. Children with uveitis need constant ophthalmic follow-up as they can have ongoing inflammation without any symptoms and minimal signs.

8 As mentioned previously, although AAU can be thought of as a distinct disease entity, uveitis itself is a common sequelae to

many ocular diseases. The combination of redness and photo-phobia is a symptom that must **never** be ignored. This is particularly true after intraocular surgery of any type when a mild uveitis may be the early sign of an endophthalmitis that can wipe out the eye in a matter of hours. Refer these patients immediately.

9 A first episode of idiopathic AAU rarely occurs in patients over the age of 60 and it is more likely to be secondary to other eye disease or very rarely part of a neoplastic process (masquerade syndrome).

Bacterial keratitis

Typical presentation

Microbial keratitis is an infection of the cornea. Bacterial keratitis is actually a rare condition and usually only occurs if the corneal defences are breached. By far the commonest risk factor is poor lens hygiene and extended wearing of contact lenses — as only soft contact lenses can be worn for long periods without discomfort they are usually implicated in bacterial keratitis.

Patients with abnormal ocular surfaces, e.g. dry eye or those with some degree of immunocompromise, are also at higher risk of bacterial keratitis.

Typical symptoms are of a unilateral, increasingly painful, injected eye that is often photophobic (secondary to the associated anterior uveitis). This description would also fit with the symptoms of acute anterior uveitis itself, but inspection of the cornea in bacterial keratitis will reveal a white/yellow corneal opacity, which is the infection itself. There may also be a hypopyon (Figure 3.4).

Principles of treatment

1 Bacterial keratitis is an ophthalmic emergency, certain organisms, e.g. *Pseudomonas aeroginosa*, can blind an eye within 24 hours.

2 Always have a high index of suspicion of a unilateral red eye in a soft contact lens wearer.

3 When referring contact lens wearers to eye casualty, tell them to take their contact lenses, contact lens case, and its fluid to the eye department. These are cultured and can help in isolating the organism.

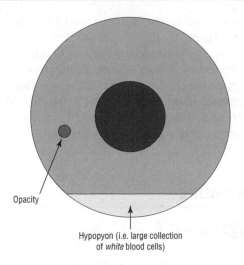

Opacity

Hypopyon (i.e. large collection
of *white* blood cells)

Figure 3.4 Corneal ulcer and hypopyon.

What you should do

1 As mentioned above, if you suspect bacterial keratitis refer the patient immediately.
2 Refer all contact lens wearers with painful, unilateral red eyes to eye casualty. Even if the cornea is clear the infected area may be too small to see without a slit-lamp or the patient may have an early *Acanthamoeba* keratitis.
3 There is no point swabbing the eye prior to referral as the pick-up rate is very low. Microbiological diagnosis is made by scraping the lesion with a sterile needle (after topical anaesthetic) and inoculating the appropriate plates. This should only be done with the magnification of a slit-lamp.
4 Treatment is with frequent (hourly) fortified antibiotic drops initially. This can be done as an outpatient or inpatient depending on the patient. The lesion is closely reviewed daily until it starts to improve, when the antibiotics are slowly reduced.
5 A variety of bacteria can be responsible. In young contact lens wearers one of the commonest and most virulent organisms is *P. aeroginosa* — this can perforate a cornea in hours. In the elderly patient streptococci and staphylococci are more common.

Episcleritis and scleritis

Typical presentation

Scleritis is an inflammatory process of the sclera, while episcleritis is an inflammatory process of the tissue overlying the sclera. Although the two conditions can look similar there are a number of features that help to separate them.

Both present as injected areas highlighted against the white sclera. These can vary in size from small raised areas to diffuse injection of the whole anterior sclera. The essential difference between the two is that scleritis is painful while episcleritis only causes a mild discomfort. Patients with scleritis are much more likely to have an associated systemic disease than do patients with episcleritis.

Principles of treatment

1 Separate episcleritis or scleritis from other causes of a red eye.
2 Separate the features of episcleritis from those of scleritis.
3 Episcleritis may not require treatment if it is painless.
4 Scleritis needs treatment and it is not uncommon for this to be systemic.
5 If the history suggests an underlying cause for the scleritis the patient will need referral to a physician — usually a rheumatologist.

How and what to do

1 When separating episcleritis and scleritis from other causes of a red eye look for certain features.
   Features not associated with episcleritis/scleritis:
   – stickiness/discharge
   – cough or cold
   – bilateral
   – corneal staining.
   Features associated with episcleritis/scleritis:
   – discrete areas of redness — sometimes slightly raised

– tender to the touch (scleritis)

2 Separating episcleritis from scleritis can often be done on the history alone:

- Episcleritis is a mild condition causing mild discomfort/ irritation and patients may well present with the red patch only.
- Episcleritis has not been shown to be persistently associated with any systemic diseases.
- Scleritis is painful — often the patients describe it as a deep, boring pain which keeps them awake at night.
- Coexisting systemic disease is reasonably common, although it is unusual for scleritis to be a presenting feature.
- The vision is invariably normal in episcleritis but may be reduced in scleritis.
- If the injected area is gently pressed after topical anaesthetic it will be very tender in those with scleritis.
- One useful manoeuvre is to instill 10% phenylephrine into the affected eye and wait for 5 minutes. The phenylephrine blanches the superficial blood vessels but not the deep. This is best viewed in natural light rather than with a pen-torch. With conjunctivitis or episcleritis, the redness will disappear, but with scleritis a deep redness will still be seen.

3 The treatment of episcleritis depends on symptoms:

- If painless, then the patient can be reassured and no treatment is required.
- If the patient is concerned by the redness try g. Isopto Frin (phenylephrine and hypromellose) qds for 1–2 weeks.
- If there is some discomfort use g. flurbiprofen 0.03% tds for 2 weeks.
- With or without treatment the vast majority will have settled within a month. If symptoms persist for more than 3 weeks refer to an ophthalmologist

4 The treatment of scleritis is very different. If it is suspected the patient must be referred immediately as it can be a sight-threatening disease. It often requires systemic steroids — or even more powerful immunosuppressants.

5 The distinction between episcleritis and scleritis is not always as simple as it appears in this topic. Pain is the major differentiating feature. If patients do have pain (whether episcleritis or scleritis) they are likely to need at least topical steroids and therefore will need ophthalmic supervision.

Herpes simplex

Typical presentation

Herpes simplex type 1 is an extremely common viral infection and usually manifests as "cold sores" on the lips. Less commonly it can infect the eye and can cause a potentially serious keratitis. Typical features are a unilateral, painful, red, photophobic eye. Important examination findings are decreased corneal sensitivity and the presence of a branching epithelial (dendritic) ulcer which shows up very well with flourescein.

Herpes simplex type 2 is a sexually transmitted disease. It is much less common in the eye but can present with an identical ocular picture.

Principles of treatment

1 There are three common situations in which ocular herpes simplex is encountered:
   - herpetic vesicles on the eyelid
   - herpes simplex conjunctivitis
   - herpes simplex keratitis (HSK).
2 HSK may occur by direct spread from the eyelid or conjunctiva or it may be as a result of reactivation of dormant virus. It does not matter as the treatment is the same.
3 Treatment is aimed at minimising the corneal damage caused by the virus and therefore reducing scarring.
4 Steroids are used with great care but never without concurrent antiviral treatment. Steroids given without antivirals suppress the immune response to the virus, causing very large corneal ulcers to form (called geographical ulcers). The possibility of HSK is one of the reasons that steroid drops should never be used on an undiagnosed red eye except by a specialist.
5 Type 2 herpes simplex is sexually acquired and can present as an ophthalmia neonatorum (conjunctivitis in the first month of life (see page 126)).
6 Although HSK is almost exclusively unilateral, it can be bilateral in atopes.
7 Patients who wear contact lenses should **never** be diagnosed as having HSK but should be referred to an eye department to rule out *Acanthamoeba* keratitis.

How and what to do

1 If herpetic lid vesicles are present on the eyelids but the patient has no ocular symptoms and the eye is quiet (i.e. the conjunctiva is not red), antivirals are not necessary. However, the patient must be warned to return immediately if the eye becomes sore, red or sensitive to the light. They should be instructed to attend the nearest eye casualty within 24 hours.

2 Most herpetic conjunctivitis is probably missed if it is not preceded by the vesicles but this is not harmful in itself. It is however important if a subsequent keratitis is missed.

3 Whether HSK arises from a preceding conjunctivitis or from reactivation of latent virus it presents with the same symptoms:
   – photophobia
   – conjunctival injection — especially around the junction of conjunctiva and cornea
   – decreased visual acuity
   – ocular pain.

4 In fact these features are not specific for HSK and are present with keratitis of any aetiology. As a general rule, keratitis of any sort makes ophthalmic referral necessary. The clues to deciding if the keratitis is herpetic are:
   – a past history of HSK
   – recent vesicles around the eyelids or mouth
   – decreased sensitivity of the cornea — demonstrated by lightly touching the cornea with a wisp of cotton wool.

5 Using g. fluorescein 2% and a blue light is mandatory in any keratitis but particularly with HSK. If the classic dendritic ulcer is present it is usually quite obvious, but in fact any epithelial disturbance in someone with known active herpetic disease needs treating with antivirals. The epithelial loss in HSK can take one of four forms (Figure 3.5):
   – punctate loss of epithelial cells
   – small isolated patches of epithelial loss
   – dendritic ulcer
   – geographical ulcer — when steroids have been used without antiviral cover.

6 Herpetic keratitis needs treatment and monitoring by an ophthalmologist. If a patient has definite herpetic conjunctivitis (e.g. secondary to lid vesicles) but **no** apparent corneal

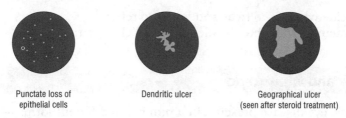

| Punctate loss of epithelial cells | Dendritic ulcer | Geographical ulcer (seen after steroid treatment) |

Figure 3.5 Different types of herpes simplex keratitis (usually seen with fluorescein).

involvement, treat with Occ. aciclovir 3% 5 times a day for 1 week and the patient should be told to return if symptoms of keratitis develop.
7 Adults diagnosed as having herpes simplex type 2, as well as ocular treatment, need referral to a genitourinary physician. Neonatal herpes simplex type 2 needs urgent referral to a paediatrician and the parents need a genitourinary opinion.

Gritty, irritable red eye

Allergy and the eye

Typical presentation

Allergic phenomena can affect the eye in a number of different ways. Typically patients complain of itch and this may be associated with red/watery eyes. They may also have a stringy discharge (which does **not** cause the eyelids to stick together in the mornings as in infective conjunctivitis). Depending on the underlying cause, sufferers may give a history of atopy, recent use of ocular medications or previous bouts of allergic eye disease.

Principles of treatment

1 Differentiate infective from allergic conjunctivitis (see also page 5).
2 Try to ascertain the underlying cause of the allergy.

3 Decide whether to treat and when to refer.
4 Remember that chronic allergies need chronic treatment.

How and what to do

Allergic eye disease presents in a number of different forms — the cause may be obvious, e.g. topical medications or a history of hay-fever, but sometimes it may not be so clear cut or may be a mixture of different allergic responses.

Allergy itself is an area that can be quite confusing and allergic eye disease is no different — there is such a profusion of different terms (often for the same condition) that it can be quite bewildering to the non-expert. This section is not a textbook description of allergic eye disease but rather a description of the commoner ways it presents:

1 The presenting symptom is itch and this is immediately sugges-tive of allergy. Ask whether it is just the lids or is it the eyes themselves? Are the eyes red? Allergic conjunctivitis can cause a thin, stringy discharge — it does not cause the eyelids to stick together as infective conjunctivitis does.
2 A history of hayfever or other forms of atopy is an extremely useful pointer in the history.
3 Use of prescribed or non-prescribed eye drops/ointments is a common cause of allergic eye disease. In fact it is usually a hyper-sensitivity to the preservatives in the medication that causes the sensitivity rather than the active drug itself.
4 Signs of ocular allergy include (non-tender) puffy lids, injected conjunctivae, papillae on the upper tarsal plate — these are diffi-cult to see without a slit-lamp unless they are very large (giant papillae). Stringy mucus can be seen in the lower fornix — it is quite unlike infective discharge as when removed from the eye it tends to elongate into long strings before it comes away from the fornix.

Types of allergic eye disease

Acute (ocular) anaphylaxis

• This is an acute allergic reaction to an antigen entering the con-junctiva.

- The reaction results in the conjunctiva rapidly filling with fluid (chemosis) causing it to expand through the lids. The patients describe this as like a "jelly coming out of the eye".
- The lids themselves often swell and can completely close the eye.
- It is very dramatic and can produce a great deal of panic in the sufferer and those around them but it quickly resolves — often by the time medical attention is given.
- It is sometimes possible to identify the allergen, e.g. if it occurs while walking in a field or playing with a dog.
- No specific treatment is required as it settles very rapidly. Reassurance that it has not harmed the eye is important.

Chronic allergic eye disease

- Some but not all of these sufferers have a history of hayfever, asthma, or eczema (sometimes called seasonal allergic conjunctivitis).
- For those who do, their systemic anti-allergic treatment may well help their ocular symptoms.
- For those with only eye disease (i.e. chronic allergic conjunctivitis) or whose systemic treatment does not alleviate their ocular symptoms local treatment is required.
- The principle of treating allergic eye disease is:
  a If possible remove the allergen.
  b Suppress the allergic response with mast cell stabilisers such as g. sodium chromoglycate 2% qds, lodoxamide 0.1% qds (Alomide), or nedocromil sodium 2% (Rapitil) qds. These are safe to use long term. If symptoms are perennial the patient should use the drops constantly. If the symptoms are seasonal they should only be used over the symptomatic period. Remember that the drops take time to have an effect so they should be started **before** the season starts. Sodium chromoglycate takes 2–4 weeks to have an effect, the other two have their effect within a week.
  c Some patients prefer vasoconstrictor-antihistamines such as antazoline (Otrivine-Antistin), but these should be avoided for very long periods as they can cause rebound hyperaemia.
  d Ocular steroids are avoided if possible because of their side effects (see page 173). They can be used for short (1–2 weeks) periods and reduced as soon as possible. Steroid drops should only be prescribed by those who have the experience and equipment to regularly check for complications.

Contact hypersensitivity

- This occurs when the conjunctiva becomes sensitised to the active ingredient or the preservative in the drop.
- Patients complain that the drop stings for longer than usual on instillation or that their eyes have become itchy and red.
- When the drug has spilt over the lid and onto the face, eczematous type skin changes can be seen on the skin under the lower lid.
- The causative agent is usually obvious and usually it can be stopped. If it needs to be continued, some drops are available in a preservative-free form. These are expensive and should only be used if strictly necessary.
- If the skin changes are particularly severe use hydrocortisone cream 1% tds to the affected area for no more than 1 week.

Allergic disorders of the lids only

- Lid swelling and itch can occur in any of the situations described above.
- Lid swelling can also occur in hayfever sufferers without any eye problems — in this case topical treatments are inappropriate.
- Allergic lid swelling and infective lid swelling are differentiated because the former is non-tender and the latter tender. It is important to separate the two as the treatment is very different — this is discussed in more detail on page 12.

Blepharitis

Typical presentation

This is an extremely common condition caused by an abnormality of the lipid-secreting meibomian glands that open onto the lid margins. Presenting symptoms are variations of itching, burning, mildly painful and watery eyes. Signs include redness along the lid margin, crusting at the base of the lashes, prominent meibomian gland orifices and a "foamy" tear film due to abnormal lipid constitution of the tears (Figure 3.6).

There appears to be a poor correlation between signs and symptoms in blepharitis, some patients present complaining of terrible symptoms but appear to have minimal signs of the disease, other patients appear to have dreadful disease but are asymptomatic.

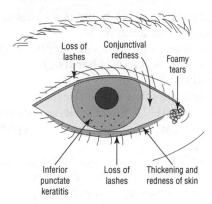

Loss of lashes
Conjunctival redness
Foamy tears
Inferior punctate keratitis
Loss of lashes
Thickening and redness of skin

Figure 3.6 Some features of blepharitis (some or all may be present).

Principles of treatment

1 The management involves both symptomatic relief and treatment of the underlying disease process.
2 Blepharitis is a chronic disease and long-term treatment is required. It is never cured as such, but symptoms wax and wane over time.
3 Look for signs of associated skin disease especially acne rosacea.
4 In the vast majority of patients, blepharitis is an annoying but benign condition. Occasionally it can be so severe that permanent corneal scarring occurs. It is probably a risk factor for endophthalmitis after intraocular surgery and so requires aggressive treatment prior to any surgery.

How and what to do

It is important to remember that patients can be very troubled by the symptoms of blepharitis.

1 Look generally at the patient, do they have any associated skin disease, e.g. seborrheic dermatitis, acne rosacea, atopic dermatitis.
2 Examine the lids, conjunctiva, cornea, and tear film:
   – With a bright light/slit-lamp examine the lid margin for redness and prominent meibomian glands. Look at the lashes — are there loose pieces of skin/debris clinging to the lashes. Look

at the tear film, is it full of bubbles — this is a good sign of meibomian gland dysfunction.

- Look at the lid itself. Patients with blepharitis tend to get chalazia (see page 83). Severe blepharitis can cause distortion and deformation of the lids.
- The conjunctivae are often injected, especially between the lids.
- Stain the cornea with 2% fluoroscein and examine with a blue light. Blepharitis can cause patchy loss of epithelium from the cornea.
- Because the lipid in the tears is deficient in patients with meibomian gland dysfunction, the tears tend to evaporate very quickly and this causes symptoms similar to those of dry eye. This is why blepharitis sufferers complain of worsening of symptoms in dry and smoky atmospheres or when reading or watching television (in these latter activities the blink rate is reduced and this means the tears are not being continually spread over the corneal surface).
- A good way of testing the tear evaporation is to look for the tear film break-up time (TFBUT). With fluorescein in, hold the eyelids open and time how long it is until the even flourescein film becomes patchy. No patches of drying should be seen within 5 seconds; if there are the patient is likely to respond well to artificial tears.

3 The most important element of the treatment is an explanation to the patient:
- What the condition is.
- That it is not sight-threatening.
- That effective treatment is available.
- That blepharitis is not curable and therefore treatment is long term.

4 Initial treatment of blepharitis:
- The patient needs to clean the eyelid margins of debris from the lashes and encourage normal meibomian function (this is sometimes called "lid hygiene"). It may be worth contacting the local eye department to see if they have any patient information leaflets on blepharitis which give instructions regarding lid hygiene techniques.
- The patient should use a mild shampoo such as Johnson's baby shampoo and dilute it to a 1:3 solution in warm water. Then using a cotton bud dipped in the shampoo, the eyelid margins should be gently scrubbed near the eye lashes. This should be repeated twice a day until symptoms improve

when the patient can then titrate the need for lid hygiene with his/her symptoms.

- Some ophthalmologists prefer to use sodium bicarbonate solution rather than baby shampoo.
- Because of the rapid tear evaporation, many blepharitis sufferers get relief from tear substitutes such as hypromellose. These should be used as required — there is no limit to the number of times they need to be used.

5 If this does not relieve symptoms:
- Not uncommonly there is secondary staphylococcal colonisation of the lid margin and it can be helpful to prescribe an antibiotic ointment to be smeared onto the lids margins, e.g. fucidic acid bd or Occ. erythromycin bd for 1 month. They should continue lid hygiene during this.
- If the patient does not respond to this or has rosacea, a prolonged course of oral antibiotics may be extremely helpful. Try oral tetracycline 250 mg bd or doxycycline 50 mg od for 3–6 months. Avoid these in children under 12, pregnant and breast-feeding women, and remember that they can cause photosensitivity.

6 Referral to an ophthalmologist is not indicated for the vast majority of patients with blepharitis; however situations in which this may be indicated include:
- When the patient remains symptomatic despite trying the above treatment for an adequate (months not weeks) length of time.
- When there is an associated skin disease (alternatively consider referral to a dermatologist).
- If there are any signs of corneal involvement.
- Children.

Note: Although this topic considers blepharitis as one diagnosis, it is really a number of overlapping conditions such as seborrheic dermatitis, meibomianitis, and demodex infection.

Conjunctivitis

Typical presentation

Infective conjunctivitis tends to present with bilateral, red, sticky eyes — patients often complain that they cannot open their eyes in the mornings because of the stickiness. The complaint is of grittiness, **not** pain.

Helpful associations include concurrent cough and cold and the presence of a pre-auricular lymph node (indicating viral or chlamydial cause). Itchiness is not a strong feature of infective conjunctivitis and, if present, then think of a purely allergic cause or if the patient has already been treated for infective conjunctivitis think of an allergy to the medication.

Principles of treatment

1 Differentiate via history and examination between infective and allergic conjunctivitis.
2 Is the patient in a high-risk group for chlamydial conjunctivitis?
3 If a bacterial conjunctivitis is suspected treat with topical antibiotics where appropriate for an adequate length of time.
4 Not everyone needs swabs.
5 Ensure strict hygiene as viral conjunctivitis can be very contagious.
6 If VA is altered this may suggest an associated keratitis and the patient needs referral.
7 Ophthalmia neonatorum is an ophthalmic emergency and needs same-day referral.

How and what to do

1 Differentiate between the different types of conjunctivitis with the history and examination:
Bacterial conjunctivitis:
 – sticky red eye
 – no lymph nodes in front of the ears (Figure 3.7)
 – no coexisting cough or cold.
Viral conjunctivitis:
 – sticky red eye
 – pre-auricular lymph nodes (Figure 3.7)
 – coexisting cough and cold.
Chlamydial conjunctivitis:
 – sticky red eye
 – pre-auricular lymph nodes
 – no coexisting cough and cold
 – may have genitourinary symptoms.

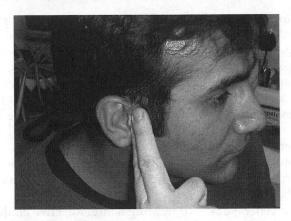

Figure 3.7 Examining for presence of pre-auricular lymph nodes in conjunctivitis.

Allergic conjunctivitis:
- itchy red eye
- no lymph nodes
- systemically well (may be atopic).

2 Bacterial conjunctivitis is treated with topical antibiotic for 1 week. Conjunctivitis that appears viral in origin is self limiting; however, most practitioners give antibiotic cream or drops in case of secondary bacterial infection, or because the patient expects it. Treatment of chlamydial conjunctivitis is outlined below.

3 The majority of ophthalmologists use chloramphenicol despite fears about (extremely rare) systemic side effects. Neomycin is a useful alternative but has a relatively high rate of contact sensitivity. Topical gentamicin, ofloxacin, tetracylines or fucidic acid can also be used.

4 Some patients prefer drops, but in the case of g. chloramphenicol they need to be used 2 hourly to be effective. Although the ointment can be slightly greasy (and so temporarily blur the vision) it is useful in that it need only be administered qds. For these reasons Occ. chloramphenicol qds is the commonest treatment for infective conjunctivitis.

5 It is seldom necessary to treat for more than 1 week, although residual symptoms may persist a little longer, e.g. a little stickiness or redness. If symptoms are not **improving** after 1 week then there may be various reasons:
- The bacteria are resistant to chloramphenicol (very rare).

- The infection is with a strain of virus that causes more prolonged infection — most often this is adenovirus.
- The patient has chlamydial conjunctivitis.
- The patient is beginning to develop an allergy to the drops.

6 The pragmatic approach is to stop all treatment and ask the patient to return in 1 week's time. The natural history of the disease will mean a further proportion of patients have improved and those that have an allergy to the medication will also have improved.

7 If symptoms do remain into this second week the patient should be referred to an eye casualty to ease both practitioner's and patient's minds.

8 This is a general guide to treating acute, infective conjunctivitis but there are certain situations that should ring alarm bells:
- Conjunctivitis within the first month of life (ophthalmia neonatorum) is a potentially blinding condition and needs urgent referral — it is dealt with below.
- Beware the young adult with unilateral or bilateral conjunctivitis, a pre-auricular lymph node, and who is resistant to treatment. Most will still have viral conjunctivitis but always ask if they have genitourinary symptoms and have a low threshold for swabbing for chlamydia.
- If lid vesicles are present at presentation, herpes simplex conjunctivitis is a possibility. Treat with Occ. aciclovir 3% 5 times a day for 1 week and strongly warn the patient to attend an eye casualty if their vision is altered (see "herpes simplex", page 113).
- If the patient is a contact lens wearer.

Instructions for the patient

1 Explain to the patient that conjunctivitis can persist for some weeks but usually lasts for only 7–10 days.

2 During this time the patient does not need regular review as this is simply increasing the chance for other patients (or yourself) of becoming cross infected.

3 However, if the patient feels the symptoms are getting worse or their vision is declining or that the treatment is making things worse (i.e. contact sensitivity) they should be told to return.

4 Conjunctivitis is usually very contagious. Patients should be told to use separate towels, pillowcases, etc. and to wash their hands. Remember to wash your hand and instruments after examining a

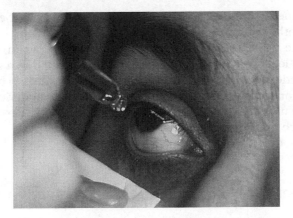

Figure 3.8 Technique for pulling down lower lid when instilling eyedrops.

patient with conjunctivitis. Alcohol swabs and air drying are adequate for instruments.

5 Do not wear contact lenses until the symptoms have settled and get a new pair of lenses and cases.

6 Instilling treatment:
   – Drops — wash hands first. Pull lower lid down, patient should be looking up, shake bottle and squeeze on drop into the lower fornix (Figure 3.8). Do not worry if more than one drop is instilled as the excess will simply run down the face.
   – Ointment/gels — wash hands first. Pull lower lid down, patient should be looking up and squeeze a fingernail length onto inner surface of the lid. Warn the patient that it will blur the vision for a few minutes

Swabs are indicated when

1 A non-viral conjunctivitis has not responded to antibiotics.
2 There is a high index suspicion for chlamydia.
3 Ophthalmia neonatarum.

How to take a swab

1 Wash your hands.
2 Swabs can be taken for viruses, bacteria, and chlamydia.
3 Make sure you use the correct swab (ask microbiologist if any doubts).

4 Anaesthetise the eye with a minimal amount of g. benoxinate (g. amethocaine has some bactericidal properties).
5 Run the tip of the swab over the lower fornix (again, with the patient looking up and the lower lid being pulled down to expose the inferior conjunctiva) once forward and backwards in both eyes, even if only one eye is affected. Use a different swab for each eye.
6 Fill the microbiology forms carefully, paying particular attention to which antibiotics have been used.
7 Wash your hands.

Treatment of chlamydial inclusion conjunctivitis

- Prescribe tetracycline 250–500 mg PO qds, or doxycycline 100 mg PO bid or erythromycin 250–500 mg PO qds for 3 weeks. Remember that tetracyclines are contraindicated for children less than 12 years, pregnant or breast-feeding women, and that they can make the user's skin photosensitive.
- Arrange for the patient to be seen in a sexually transmitted diseases clinic and inform the patient that their sexual partners will need to be treated. Explain to the patient the potential seriousness of the condition and the importance of attending the genitourinary clinic. This can, of course, be potentially devastating for the patient or their partner — be sure of the diagnosis before breaking the news.
- Ask the patient to be seen in an eye casualty department in 1 week's time.

Ophthalmia neonatorum

- This is a conjunctivitis within the first month of life and is an ophthalmic emergency.
- Same-day ophthalmic opinion is mandatory.
- Urgent swabs are taken for gram staining, bacterial culture and sensitivity, chlamydia and herpes simplex type 2.
- Treatment is with systemic and intensive topical antibiotics.
- A paediatric opinion is also required as respiratory complications can occur.
- If chlamydia, gonococcal or herpetic infections are found, the parents will need a genitourinary opinion.
- It is a notifiable disease.

Dry eye

Typical presentation

Patients usually complain of chronic, itchy, burning eyes. Symptoms tend to be worse in dry atmospheres, e.g. centrally heated or air-conditioned rooms or when reading or watching television when the blink rate is reduced. Occasionally patients volunteer that they find it difficult to cry when upset or when peeling onions. The condition may or may not present with an associated systemic disease.

Signs are variable and depend on the severity of the tear deficit.

Principles of treatment

1 The majority of cases are idiopathic but it is important to be aware of the systemic associations of dry eye. It is rare for any of these systemic diseases to present with dry eye and the diagnosis is usually well established. Therefore, unless there are other symptoms a patient with dry eye does not need further investigation. The systemic associations of dry eye are listed below.
2 The ocular surface needs constant bathing in tears to maintain its integrity, thus the treatment of dry eye is tear replacement.
3 Abnormalities of the ocular surface increase the risk of microbial keratitis.

How and what to do

1 Take a full history looking for symptoms of associated systemic disease.
2 Check the visual acuity, allow the patient time for this as they often need to blink frequently.
3 Examine the lids for signs of blepharitis as this can often coexist with dry eye and is important to treat in its own right.
4 Using a pen-torch and magnifier or ophthalmoscope set to +10 or a slit-lamp, look at the tear meniscus of the lower lid. In patients with dry eye it is often almost completely absent.The bright lustre of the cornea is often absent.
5 Instill 2% fluorescein into the lower fornix and using a blue filter:
   – Examine the tear meniscus.

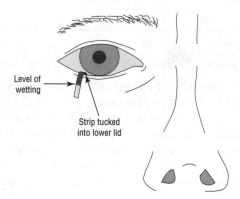

Level of wetting

Strip tucked into lower lid

Figure 3.9 Schirmer's test.

- Look for irregularities of the corneal epithelium (caused by patchy loss of epithelium).
- Look for debris in the tear film (dead and dying epithelial cells and mucus).
- Look for staining areas on the (usually medial) conjunctiva — a good sign of dry eyes.

6 Schirmer's test should really be used as a **confirmation** of the diagnosis as it is relatively non-specific. The principle is simple:
  - A strip of filter paper is placed in the lower fornix overlapping the lid (Figure 3.9).
  - The more tears that are produced the higher up the filter paper that becomes damp.
  - It can be performed with or without topical anaesthetic as long as you are consistent.
  - Most ophthalmologists use one drop of g. benoxinate as it is more comfortable for the patient, and reflex tearing from the irritation of the paper itself is removed.
  - The Schirmer filter paper is placed between the inner and middle third of the eyelid.
  - The patient is asked to gently shut the eyes for 5 minutes, after which the height of wetting of the paper is measured in millimetres (there is a measuring scale on the box containing the papers).
  - After 5 minutes, wetting of less than 5 mm is highly suggestive of tear deficiency (in the context of other findings). More than 15 mm in 5 minutes suggests normal tear production.

7 Treatment involves tear replacement and treatment of any associated blepharitis. The treatment of blepharitis is dealt with on pages 118–121.

8 The mainstay of dry eye treatment is artificial tears:
   - These can be given as often as the patient feels necessary, which can be a number of times per hour.
   - They all really perform the same function and therefore it is best to start with the cheaper ones such as hypromellose and instruct patients to use it as many times as required to reduce their symptoms.
   - If they do not get relief its worth trying different types, e.g. Liquifilm Tears, g. sodium chloride, or Tears Naturale.
   - Viscotears are preferred by some patients as they are more viscous than hypromellose and therefore their effects last longer.
   - If excess mucus is a problem a combination of acetylcysteine (a mucolytic) and hypromellose can help (e.g. Ilube).
   - If the patient is arthritic, a pharmacist can often help with specially designed devices that help with drop instillation.
   - If a patient initially gets relief from a drop but later finds it increasingly irritating **and** itchy it is likely that he/she has developed an allergy to the preservative in the drops. It is worth trying a course of preservative-free drops. If these do not give relief change the drop.
   - Many patients with dry eyes do not like ointment as it smears their vision. However it is useful last thing at night, especially if the patient has incomplete lid closure when asleep (lagophthalmos).
9 The majority of patients with dry eyes do not need ophthalmologic referral but certain groups do:
   - No relief after three drops of different types have been tried.
   - If there is sudden increase in discomfort, redness or decrease in vision the patient needs urgent referral (patients with dry eyes are at increased risk of microbial keratitis).
   - If patients are putting in drops so often that it is affecting their lives. In these circumstances the ophthalmologist may decide to block up the lacrimal punctae to reduce tear drainage.
   - If patients want to continue wearing contact lenses.

Some systemic associations of dry eyes

- Collagen vascular diseases, e.g. Wegener's granulomatosis, systemic lupus erythematosus (SLE), Sjögren's syndrome, rheumatoid arthritis.

- Conjunctival scarring, e.g. post Stevens–Johnson syndrome, post chemical injury to the conjunctiva, ocular pemphigoid.
- Drugs, e.g. antihistamines, anticholinergics, oral contraceptives.

Eyelash nits (phthiriasis palpebrarum)

Typical presentation

Phthiriasis palpebrarum is infestation of the eyelids with the pubic crab louse, *Phthirus pubis*. This presents with an often prolonged history of bilateral blepharitis with the major symptoms usually itchy, crusty lids that do not improve with topical antibiotics. There may or may not be an associated conjunctivitis.

Close examination of the lashes, especially with some form of magnification, readily reveals the organisms and their eggs.

Principles of treatment

1 The diagnosis is often missed simply because it is not thought of, but it must be in the differential diagnosis of apparently recent onset of blepharitis in those who are sexually active.
2 As well as treating the lashes, the patient needs referral to a genitourinary physician for treatment and contact tracing.

How and what to do

1 A number of different treatments have been advocated for phthiriasis palpebrarum, including cryotherapy and argon laser ablation. A mainstay of treatment was Occ. physostigmine 0.25% but this is not now commercially available.
2 Current treatment options:
   - Manual removal of organisms and eggs from the lashes using forceps. This is time consuming and very difficult in children.
   - Petroleum jelly can be smothered on the lashes twice a day for 8 days, but it does not kill the eggs.
   - Aqueous malathion lotion 1% applied carefully to the lashes using a cotton bud and washed off with saline after 5

minutes. This is repeated 2 days later. This appears to be effective and acceptable to patients. Avoid getting any of the lotion into the patient's eyes and **do not** use the 0.5% formulation as this contains alcohol and irritates the eye. Malathion 1% is now probably the treatment of choice but it does not have a product licence for the treatment of lash infestation.
  – Ivermectin (an antihelminthic) may be the treatment of choice in the future.
3 Refer the patient to a genitourinary physician who will prescribe treatment (which involves the whole body) and will organise contact tracing. If the patient is a child it is important to discuss the situation with a paediatrician.

Things that go "ouch!" in the night

There are a trio of conditions which result in epithelial disturbance when the patient is asleep. Typically the patient feels pain or discomfort on waking each morning, but the pain settles over a few hours. Examination of the eye often takes place some hours later, when the epithelium has healed — thus the diagnosis usually needs to be made on the history.

Recurrent epithelial erosion syndrome (RES)

Typical presentation

This is a not infrequent problem for patients but most non-ophthalmologists are usually unaware of its existence. Patients complain of sudden ocular pain on waking. They will also, if questioned, usually give a history of a traumatic corneal abrasion weeks, months or years beforehand.

Principles of treatment

1 The underlying cause is a prolonged abnormality of epithelial attachment to its basement membrane.
2 If the abrasion is still present treat as usual (see pages 139–144).

3 Ointment is used to protect the abnormal epithelium during sleep. This needs to be continued for months.

RES presents with a typical history:

1 Prior history (weeks, months or years before) of a traumatic abrasion.
2 During sleep the epithelium breaks down and the patient experiences a sudden onset of pain on opening the eyelids.
3 The pain lasts until the abrasion heals (usually a few hours).
   - The immediate management is as for a corneal abrasion, although by the time the patient presents the abrasion may have already healed. So if the **history** is suggestive, treatment is initiated.
   - Long-term management involves protecting the abnormal area of epithelium during sleep with a lubricating eye ointment (e.g. Occ. Simplex) or hypertonic saline ointment (e.g. Occ. sodium chloride 5%). This should be instilled very last thing at night for at least 3 months.
   - If this fails, refer to an ophthalmologist but continue with the ointment in the mean time.

Floppy eyelid syndrome

Patients complain of irritation, redness and discharge on awakening (not pain as in recurrent abrasion syndrome). Patients are typically males and overweight.

1 The underlying problem is thought to be an excessively lax upper lid that is easily everted. The lid can evert spontaneously during sleep, leading to exposure of the upper lid conjunctiva.

2 The diagnosis is often missed as most practitioners are unaware of the existence of the syndrome.

How and what to do

1 Take a good history — this is the key to the diagnosis. Is there an association of symptoms in the morning? How long have the symptoms been present?
2 Examine the lids: it is usually possible to easily evert the upper lid with minimal force.
3 Try to exclude other causes of chronic conjunctivitis, e.g. contact lens related (contact lens wear), vernal conjunctivitis (itchy eyes with a seasonal variation and discharge, usually young men), blepharitis, or mucus fishing syndrome.*
4 Treatment involves keeping the cornea lubricated and protected during sleep:
   - Use lubricating ointment last thing at night e.g. Occ. Simplex or Lacri-Lube.
   - If this does not help tape the lid shut at night.
   - If symptoms persist, the patient can be referred to an ophthalmologist for surgery to tighten the lids.
   - Help the patient to lose weight.

Nocturnal lagophthalmos

Typical presentation

Lagophthalmos is incomplete closure of the eyelids and can result in corneal exposure, drying, and infection. Mild cases may only cause symptoms at night because the small area of exposed corneal epithelium dries out. In the morning, the patient has discomfort until the epithelium heals.

It can occur in a number of otherwise normal individuals or as a result of lid abnormalities (e.g. after injury — including surgery),

---

* Mucus fishing syndrome is caused by the sufferer's attempts to remove mucus strands from his/her conjunctivae. This tends to cause mechanical damage to the conjunctivae, further mucus production and a vicious cycle is established. Treatment is to stop fishing — the syndrome is often overlooked as a cause of chronic conjunctivitis.

facial palsies or as a result of globe proptosis (e.g. thyroid eye disease).

Principles of treatment

1 Again the diagnosis is often missed, particularly suspect it when the patient has had eyelid surgery, injury, or thyroid eye disease.
2 Treat with lubricants last thing at night.

How and what to do

1 The history should be much as described above. Ask about previous eyelid problems or history of thyroid problems.
2 Examine the eye for signs of proptosis (see page 45).
3 Look at the lids, are there any signs of notching or distortion of the lid?
4 Ask the patient to close their eyes tightly — is there an obvious gap between the lids?
5 It is important to look for the Bell's phenomenon. This is the reflex that protects the eye when the lids are closed and results in the eye rotating upwards. If you manually hold the lids open and ask the patient to shut their eyes tightly you should see the eye disappearing upwards until the cornea cannot be seen. If Bell's phenomenon is not present (i.e. most of the cornea can still be seen), it means that the cornea is at a greater risk of severe exposure.
6 Instill 2% fluorescein and examine the corneal epithelium with a blue light. It is likely to be normal as the epithelium heals quickly.
7 Management:
   – If there appears to be no underlying cause and the patient has a good Bell's phenomenon, prescribe Occ. Simplex last thing at night for 3 months.
   – If this does not work, instruct the patient (or their partner) to tape the lid shut at night.
   – If the patient has a poor Bell's phenomenon begin lubricants and refer them to an ophthalmologist.
   – If the patient has an obvious underlying cause, e.g. lid position abnormality or proptosis, refer them to an ophthalmologist.

Trauma

Chemical and thermal burns

Typical presentation

Chemical and thermal burns to the eye are a common occurrence. Most are uncomfortable but heal rapidly and without sequelae, but some can be sight threatening. Although all ocular burns need full assessment, generally alkaline burns cause more damage than do acid or thermal.

Presentation is usually obvious and the patient is usually in great distress. Chemical burns are one of the few situations where treatment should begin before an adequate history is taken, i.e. if patients present and say that a chemical has entered their eye, they should have their eyes irrigated (washed out) immediately. Further history and examination can be carried out later.

Principles of treatment

1 Irrigate first, ask questions later.
2 Take a full history and examine the eye carefully — a white (i.e. non-injected) eye can indicate that all the conjunctival vasculature has been destroyed (but only in the context of the seriousness of the injury, of course).
3 When in doubt refer to an eye unit.
4 CS gas injuries are treated differently to other chemical burns and should not be irrigated.

How and what to do

1 The patient is often in great pain. Instill g. benoxinate into the conjunctiva to relieve this. Often there is tight blepharospasm (lid closure). To overcome this, gently but firmly pull the lids apart and get a second person to drop the benoxinate in. The anaesthetic will sting, but within 30 seconds the patient will get relief; at this point add more benoxinate and keep on instilling it until it no longer stings. Unless there is nothing else available, do not use g. amethocaine as it can be toxic to an already damaged corneal epithelium.

2 Once the patient is more comfortable the eye needs to be irrigated. This involves a high flow of fluid over the conjunctiva
and cornea to wash out/dilute any remaining chemical or to
rapidly cool the ocular tissues with a thermal burn. In alkaline
injuries the alkali can penetrate deep into the eye and the irrigation has a dialysis effect on the intraocular pH:

– The irrigating substance is not important. Ideally use a 1 litre
bag of normal saline attached to an IV giving set, open it up
to maximum flow, and irrigate the eye. The patient's chest
can be covered with a protective cover — a plastic bin-liner
tied around the neck will suffice for this, collect the excess
fluid in a bowl held under the eye, e.g. an (unused) vomit
bowl. It is important that the patient can bend the head
back, so a reclining chair or barber-type chair is ideal. Run
at least 1 litre over the eye. The set-up is illustrated in Figure
3.10.

– If bags of saline are not available, fill a jug full of tap water and
pour it slowly into the eye. If even that is not available fill a sink
full of water, get the patient to put their whole face into the
water and slowly open and close the eye. This is a surprisingly

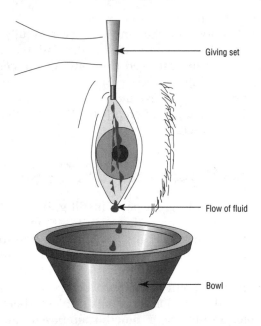

Figure 3.10 Proper method of ocular irrigation after chemical or thermal burn.

effective method, although it is wise to let the patient breathe once in a while!
- While irrigating, evert the upper lid (see pages 156–157) and wash it. If lime or concrete has gone into the eye it often gets caught under the upper lid, if there are large pieces remove them with forceps.
- Do not forget to irrigate the other eye if there is any question of damage to it — if necessary irrigate both simultaneously.

3 Once the irrigation has finished and the patient is comfortable take a more detailed history (bearing in mind that there may be legal issues if the patient was assaulted).
- What were the circumstances of the injury?
- What was the substance involved? In accidental situations the patient may well have brought the substance with them (if there is not a full explanation of the contents of a product, ring the nearest poisons unit for advice).
- It is helpful to know not only the substance involved but its concentration and how much of the substance appeared to go into the eye.

4 Ascertaining the type, concentration and amount of the substance is important because it indicates the potential for damage to the eye, e.g. a small splash of dilute acid is unlikely to cause a great deal of eye damage, but a fine spray of concentrated ammonia may well. Alkalis can penetrate tissues relatively easily to reach the anterior chamber and lens while acid and thermal injuries coagulate tissue and therefore form a barrier to further penetration. This is important to bear in mind when deciding on the need for referral. In general:
- Alkalis cause more damage than do acids, which in turn do more damage than thermal injuries.
- Of the alkalis, ammonia and sodium hydroxide are potentially the most dangerous.
- Of the acids, the lower the pH the more potentially damaging they are.

5 Although the above is useful in deciding the potential for injury, all chemical/thermal injuries **must** be examined carefully, as in the right circumstances they all have the potential for serious eye damage:
- Visual acuity — suspicious if markedly down (but serious injury can be still have occurred if the vision is good).
- Examine the lids — if there are skin or lid margin burns the patient will need ophthalmic referral even without eye damage. If there are major facial burns refer to plastic surgery.

- Examine the conjunctiva — if it is injected this actually may be a good sign as it indicates that the injury has not destroyed the conjunctival blood vessels. If the eye is not injected then look to see if you can see **any** conjunctival vessels — if not refer immediately. Also use the information from the history, if someone has had concentrated ammonia squirted in their eye it is unlikely that the eye will be completely white unless the vessels have been destroyed.
- Look at the cornea — does it have its normal bright appearance or is it dull/cloudy? If you cannot see the iris clearly it is likely that the cornea has been seriously damaged.
- Put a drop of 2% fluorescein into the eye. Care is again needed here, fluorescein shows up corneal abrasions because it pools in the base of the abrasion forming a thicker layer of fluorescein than the surrounding epithelium. The abrasion shows up because of the **difference** in amount of stain between the abrasion and the epithelium. This means that if all the epithelium is lost the cornea will stain uniformly, i.e. it looks normal.
- If the pupil is fixed this is extremely suspicious of severe damage.

6 It is important to have a low threshold for ophthalmic referral if the injury was potentially serious or there are significant findings on examination.

7 If, however, the injury appears mild prescribe Occ. chloramphenicol qds for 1 week. It is worth reviewing the patient the following day — if the injury was mild the patient will be comfortable. If pain persists, the vision is down or there are any new examination findings, refer the patient to eye casualty.

8 Measuring the pH of the conjunctiva is often advocated in chemical injury prior to and after irrigation. In fact this often adds little information, the pH of the conjunctiva may well not be representative of the pH of the anterior chamber, which is where the damage is being done. All injuries should be fully irrigated regardless of the pH of the conjunctiva.

Detergent injuries

- Splashing detergents or liquid soaps into the eye is quite common.
- Some can be highly alkaline and therefore irrigation is required, although serious corneal damage is rare.

- Examination usually shows a punctate epithelial loss. Prescribe Occ. chloramphenicol qds for 3 days.

CS gas injuries

CS gas (tear gas, mace) causes an intense irritation of the eyes that lasts for around 15 minutes, although there have been some cases of prolonged irritation.

Prolonged ocular irritation is treated differently from other chemical injuries:

- Assess the whole patient — are there any respiratory symptoms, are there large areas of burned skin?
- Residual CS gas on the victim represents a hazard to the attending staff and therefore the patient should be examined in a well-ventilated room.
- The extent of eye damage depends on how near the victim was to the spray when it was discharged.
- Eye irrigation is **not** indicated but the eyes are treated by blowing **air** into them, allowing the gas to vaporise. This can be done using a blow dryer or a heated fan — staff must avoid getting into the draught of this.
- The patient's eyes should be examined for any evidence of ocular damage as discussed above and referred if necessary.

Corneal abrasion

Typical presentation

Patients tends to give a history of a minor injury to the affected eye, e.g. when brushing hair, from a child's finger or a piece of paper or plant when gardening. Corneal abrasions are very painful and patients often present in great distress.

Principles of treatment

1 If the patient is in distress then immediately instill a few drops of local anaesthetic such as g. benoxinate or amethocaine until the patient is comfortable. Corneal abrasions can be very painful but

because they are superficial the anaesthetic often has a very good effect, making examination much easier and doing wonders for the doctor–patient relationship.

2 As ever, make sure you have checked the visual acuity — again this may be easier after some topical anaesthetic.

3 If the patient has not given a history of trauma begin to think of other causes of corneal abrasion.

4 **Always ask whether the patient wears contact lenses.** Abrasions in contact lens wearers must be treated with caution, i.e. all should be followed up in an eye department.

5 Like any epithelial loss on the body, covering the area will make it more comfortable and more likely to heal. For the cornea this can be done with a well-fitting eye pad.

6 Because the epithelium has been broached, like any other lesion there is the possibility of secondary infection. Therefore topical antibiotics are used and prolonged padding is avoided.

7 Children who are 7 years of age or under should not be padded if at all possible.

How and what to do

1 When the patient is comfortable and can fully open their eyes take the history — was there history of trauma? Is the patient a contact lens wearer?

2 Before commencing the examination make sure the patient is comfortable:
   - It is worth waiting for the patient to feel comfortable and adding more anaesthetic rather than pushing the patient quickly into the examination.
   - Patients who have an abrasion are sometimes more comfortable if the room lights are dimmed.

3 The abrasion can be examined with or without a slit-lamp (this is detailed in Section 2), but remember:
   - Abrasions are best seen by using g. fluorescein 2%.
   - There is no point using fluorescein without some sort of blue light source — this is available on the slit-lamp (see p. 53) and some pen-torches have a blue filter on their end.
   - Always use a source of magnification if available, e.g. turn the ophthalmoscope to +10D (i.e. the red numbers).
   - A Woods light can be useful for spotting abrasions — especially in young children who may only allow you a quick glimpse.

Instill the fluorescein 2%, turn the room lights off and the Woods light on. When the patient opens his/her eyes the abrasion often lights up like a beacon.

4 If there is not a definite history of ocular trauma but an abrasion is present, look for other possible causes:
   - Check that the eye lashes are not turned inwards.
   - Check for a subtarsal foreign body (see pages 156–157).
   - Check for recurrent corneal abrasion (see below)
   - Check for floppy eyelid syndrome (see pages 132–133).
   - If the patient is a contact lens wearer refer them to an eye unit the same day.
   - When using the slit-lamp it is useful to document the size of the abrasion as this can be used as a guide to improvement as the abrasion heals. Measure along the longest axis of the lesion and the one perpendicular to it.

5 **Management.** There are two schools of thought regarding the treatment of corneal abrasions:
   - Some ophthalmologists prefer to pad the eye as this reduces lid movement over the abrasion, allowing it to heal and allowing greater comfort.
   - Others feel padding is unnecessary and that abrasions heal just as well with topical antibiotics and cycloplegics.

Which method you prefer depends on your experience, although asking the patient's preference (and whether they are driving) is often helpful.

Padding

a The technique of eye padding is described below and in Figure 3.11.

b Although a number of ophthalmologists may disagree, it is often safest (as far as secondary infection is concerned) not to pad an eye for more than 24 hours.

c It is important to continue the antibiotic, e.g. Occ. chloramphenicol qds for 1 week.

d **Do not pad** patients with contact lens induced abrasion but refer them to an eye department, where they need daily follow up.

Non-padding

a These patients also need antibiotic cover and ointment is often more comfortable than drops.

b Occ. chloramphenicol can be used every 2 hours for the first 24 hours and then qds for a further week.

c The rationale of cycloplegics (i.e. iris dilators) is that they prevent painful ciliary spasm which can occur with any corneal trauma.

d G. cyclopentolate 1% tds or g. homatropine 1% od for 48 hours can be used for the more uncomfortable abrasions. G. atropine is not a good idea as its effects last long after the abrasion has healed.

e If the abrasion is small and the patient needs to drive or get back to work they usually decline padding and cycloplegic. Give them Occ. chloramphenicol 2 hourly for 24 hours and then qds for a further week and explain to them that they are going to be uncomfortable for 12–24 hours.

- Tell the patient that they will have some pain in 15–20 minutes as the anaesthetic wears off, and if this is troublesome to take 1 g of paracetamol stat.
- **Never** give the patient topical anaesthetics to take away as they prevent epithelial healing and can in fact cause further epithelial loss.
- Do not pad children under 7 years of age as there is a small risk of unmasking a squint or even of causing amblyopia.
- The instructions given to the patient depend on the size of the abrasion:

Small abrasions

- Remove eye patch after 24 hours.
- Use antibiotic ointment qds for 7 days.
- If a patch was not used then use the dilating drops for 24–48 hours and use the ointment for 7 days.
- Return if the eye is uncomfortable after the pad is removed or if the redness increases or if the vision worsens.
- If the patient wears contact lenses ask them to see their optician before resuming contact lens wear.

Large abrasions

- Treat initially as described above but ask the patient to return the next day.
- Review symptoms, visual acuity and size of the abrasion the following day and repeat until the abrasion is almost healed.
- If it is not healing, the eye becomes more injected or painful, or the vision drops, refer to an ophthalmologist immediately.

In either case the patient should be warned not to go swimming until the abrasion has healed — in case of secondary infection.

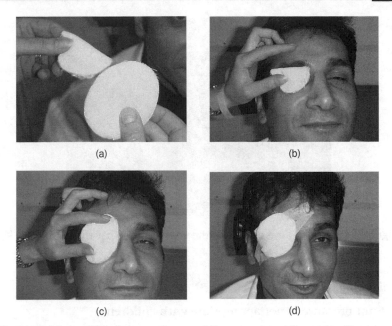

(a) (b)

(c) (d)

Figure 3.11 (a–d) Technique of eye padding — see text for explanation.

Padding the eye

To apply a double eye pad:

1 Ask the patient to shut both eyes.
2 Fold a pad in half (Figure 3.11a).
3 Press it firmly against the eyelid, asking the patient or nurse to hold it in place (Figure 3.11b).
4 Place a second unfolded pad on top (Figure 3.11c).
5 Tape this second pad to the skin (Figure 3.11d).
6 Ask the patient if the eye feels shut and is comfortable under the pad — if not repeat.

Instilling drops into the uncooperative patient

If the patient is in discomfort they reflexly close their eyelids making it difficult to instill drops (Figure 3.12).

Adults

You can usually, with firm pressure, prise open the lids and ask an assistant to instill the drops.

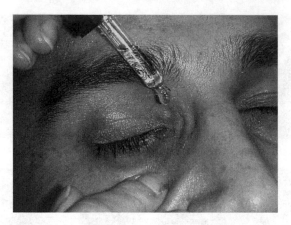

Figure 3.12 Instilling eye drops into the uncooperative patient.

Children

1 Firm pressure is not appropriate with children.
2 Lie the child on their back.
3 Place the drop on the inner canthus (Figure 3.12).
4 After a few seconds the child will open the eye and the drop will drip into the eye automatically.
5 Remember to be patient.

It can be useful to use proxymetacaine (Ophthaine) drops in children as it causes much less stinging than other topical anaesthetics.

Recurrent epithelial erosion syndrome

This is a frequent problem for patients but most non-ophthalmologists are usually unaware of its existence.

The underlying cause is a prolonged abnormality of epithelial attachment to its basement membrane, and it presents with a typical history:

• Prior history (weeks, months or years before) of a traumatic abrasion.
• During sleep the epithelium breaks down and the patient experiences a sudden onset of pain on opening the eyelids.
• The pain lasts until the abrasion heals (usually a few hours).

Management

- The immediate management is as for a corneal abrasion, although by the time they present the abrasion may have already healed. If the **history** is suggestive, treatment is indicated.
- Long-term management involves protecting the abnormal area of epithelium during sleep with a lubricating eye ointment (e.g. Occ. Simplex) or hypertonic saline ointment (e.g. Occ. sodium chloride 5%). This should be instilled very last thing at night for at least 3 months.
- If this fails, refer to an ophthalmologist but continue with the ointment in the meantime.

Corneal foreign body

Typical presentation

Presentation is usually fairly obvious as the patient gives a history of something entering their eye and subsequent discomfort. Examination usually readily reveals a foreign body (FB).

It is important to get a full history so that the force of the FB entering the eye can be judged. FBs that result from metal striking metal (e.g. hammer and chisel) are notorious for causing the FB to enter the eye itself (called an intraocular foreign body or IOFB). If there is any reason to suspect an IOFB plain X-rays of the orbit need to be taken.

Occasionally patients present who have given no history of a FB injury but have a sore, red eye and examination reveals a corneal FB — these are dealt with in the same way.

Principles of treatment

1 Have you precisely defined the nature of the injury (e.g. hammer and chisel, windblown)?
2 Has the **possibility** of an intraocular foreign body crossed your mind (see page 186 for guidance on this and indications to X-ray)?
3 Explain what you intend to do — many people are surprisingly fearful of this procedure.

4 Anaesthetise the eye as fully as possible before you start — you
 may not get a second chance.
5 Position the patient and yourself comfortably and safely.
6 Always look under the upper lid for a subtarsal foreign body (see
 "Subtarsal foreign bodies", pages 156–157) even if a corneal FB is
 found.

How and what to do

Take a full history of the injury and any visual symptoms since. If
the patient feels that his/her vision has changed, assessment by
an ophthalmologist will be needed. The external eye needs careful
examination using magnification and illumination (see Section 2).
Once the FB has been located follow the instructions below:

1 **Anaesthesia:**
 – G. benoxinate stings less than g. amethocaine but provides
  slightly less anaesthesia.
 – If available, use a few drops of benoxinate to begin the anaesthesia and when the stinging has passed deepen it with the
  amethocaine.
 – Continue to add amethocaine until further instillation only
  produces a feeling of slight **cold** rather than stinging.
2 **Instrument:**
 – The most popular instrument for removing corneal FBs is an
  ordinary venesection needle as they are easily available and sterile.
 – Many people use a green hubbed needle (21 gauge) but in fact
  an orange hub (25 gauge) is just as good and allows more
  precise movements.
 – The drawback to using the needle is that they are too small to
  hold easily. The ideal position is to hold the needle like a pen.
  To do this attach a 2-ml syringe onto the needle as this makes
  it a comfortable size and weight. A cotton bud can also be
  rammed into the hub of the needle to give the same balance
  and can be useful to brush away the FB.
3 **Positioning:**
 Positioning of yourself and the patient is vital. Whatever equipment you are using it is extremely important for both you and
 the patient to be comfortable — neither of you should be
 making any sudden or involuntary movements.
  The principle is to remove as much as possible of the FB
 without perforating the cornea. By positioning your hand and

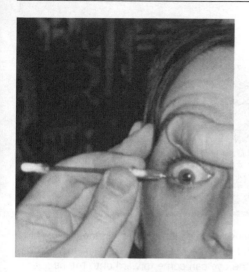

Figure 3.13 Technique for removing a foreign body without a slit-lamp. Note the hand firmly placed on the forehead to prevent forward movement. The thumb is used to hold the lid open. Note also the approach of the needle is from the side attempting to keep the plane of the needle in front of the cornea until the FB is engaged.

the patient's eye appropriately you can reduce the chance of this considerably.

Removing the FB without a slit-lamp:

- The inexperienced may first try and irrigate the FB with normal saline (see pages 136–137 for method) to dislodge it.
- Alternatively moisten a cotton bud with saline and try to gently tease the FB from the cornea. If this is not successful you will need to use a needle.
- Use the non-dominant hand to hold the eyelid open and prevent the patient moving forward onto the needle by placing the palm of your hand above the eye, and use your thumb to hold the upper lid open (Figure 3.13). Holding the needle in your dominant hand approach the eye from the side, keeping the **plane of the needle in front of the cornea**, and instruct the patient to keep looking **forward**.

With a slit-lamp:

- Make sure that the patient's head is completely forward in the lamp, i.e. their forehead is pushed against the upper plastic band (see Section 2). This means that it is very difficult for the patient to move forward onto the needle.
- Position your hand at the side of the head — you will probably require some elbow support for this — so that the **plane of the needle is in front of the cornea** (see Figure 3.14). It is very important that the patient looks **forward**.

4 *Removal*:

- Once positioned and the needle is ready, engage the top of the

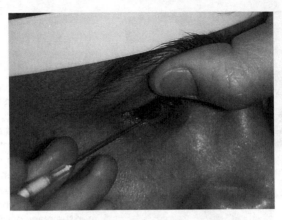

Figure 3.14 Technique for removing a foreign body with a slit-lamp. Note: the patient's head is against the band and the needle is in front of the cornea, therefore neither the patient nor the eye can come forward onto the needle.

FB and see if it brushes off easily (try this with a cotton bud to start if you prefer).
- Most will not, therefore using small sweeps gently undermine the FB piece by piece — don't worry about the pieces, the tears will wash them away.
- Remove as much of the FB as you feel comfortable with. If you or the patient feel tired stop for a rest. If the patient is feeling some pain stop and put more anaesthetic in.
5 Rust rings tend to cause some worry as they are often difficult to remove. It may be possible to remove them at one sitting but it is often better to pad the eye and try again in 24–48 hours' time when they are often very soft and easy to remove. You can either do this yourself or refer them to an eye department.
6 After removing the FB instill Occ. chloramphenicol into the eye and double pad it as you now have a corneal abrasion (see page 143 if you do not know how pad an eye). The patient can remove the pad 12–24 hours later and need not return unless they have some residual discomfort. The exception to this is if you have left a rust ring, when they should use Occ. chloramphenicol qds until review in 24–48 hours' time.
7 Instructions to the patient should be:
- Return if the eye remains uncomfortable after the pad is removed (especially if it is sensitive to the light as this usually indicates that there is residual FB).

- There will be some pain after 15–20 minutes as the anaesthetic wears off and if this is troublesome to take 1 g of paracetamol stat.
- If the patient is returning for rust removal, make sure they know how to use the Occ. chloramphenicol and that they know when and where they need to return to.

Dog bites

Typical presentation

The history is usually obvious. The dog's (or in fact any animal's) teeth, nails or claws can tear the lower lid or teeth can inflict puncture injuries to the lids or sometimes the globe itself.

Principles of treatment

1 Ascertain the extent of the injury to the lids.
2 Does it involve the lacrimal apparatus (i.e. the tear ducts and sac, situated at the medial canthus)?
3 Rule out globe perforation.
4 Cover the patient for secondary infections and tetanus.

How and what to do

1 Take a full history of the injury. Was there any associated injuries elsewhere?
2 Certain injuries need ophthalmic assessment and repair:
   - If the lid has been avulsed.
   - If the injury involves the lid margin.
   - If the injury is near the lacrimal drainage apparatus (i.e. the medial canthus).
   - If there is **any** signs of eye damage (including any change in vision).
   - If the lid injury is full thickness
Refer to eye casualty as soon as possible if any of these are present or you are worried. Tell the patient not to eat or drink as these injuries are best repaired under general anaesthetic.

3 If none of the above apply, clean the wound with iodine or chlorhexadine and remove any particulate matter. Steri-strip or stitch the wound edges if required.

4 Prescribe augmentin 1 tablet tds or erythromycin 500 mg qds for 1 week. Additionally give metronidazole 500 mg tds to cover anaerobes.

5 If the patient has not had a tetanus booster within 10 years give a booster.

6 Instruct the patient to return if the wound becomes inflamed.

Lid and orbit injuries

Lid injuries

Typical presentation

The typical presentation of eyelid injuries is usually obvious. The trauma may vary from punches or kicks to glass objects to animal paws.

Principles of treatment

1 Rule out damage to the globe itself.

2 Once you have done this the lid injury needs to be assessed.

3 Certain lid injuries should only be repaired by ophthalmologists — a poor repair can put the globe at risk.

4 Decide if antibiotics or tetanus prophylaxis are required.

How and what to do

1 Take a history of the trauma. Was it an assault? What with? Glass? Was the lid caught by a ring? Was the injury caused by an animal's paw (see "Dog bites", page 149)? Has the vision been affected? Did the patient lose consciousness at any time?

2 Examine:
   - The visual acuity.
   - Eye movements.
   - Look for a hyphaema (blood in the anterior chamber (see Figure 3.17, p. 161)) and for a fixed pupil (sign of blunt trauma).

- Add fluorescein 2% and with a blue light look for areas of corneal abrasion or epithelial loss.
- Dilate the pupil and check the fundus if possible.
- If there is any sign of ocular damage pad the eye and refer to an ophthalmologist immediately.

3 Blunt trauma to the lids can make them swell up quite quickly — from a combination of fluid and haemorrhage. This can close the lids completely and appear to make ocular examination impossible. In fact gentle but firm pressure will always open the lids enough for a superficial examination of the eye to be made. If this is difficult or if there is obvious ocular damage, again refer to an ophthalmologist.

4 Lid injuries are usually obvious — it sometimes helps to assess them more easily if they are cleaned with normal saline or some iodine diluted 50:50 with normal saline. The first and most important question to ask is "does the injury affect the eyelid margin?" If it does, it will need to be sutured by an ophthalmologist. If lid margin injuries are not sutured correctly then there may not be complete coverage of the cornea, allowing drying and possible secondary infection. Other indications for ophthalmic referral:
- If the lid has been avulsed laterally or medially or has been torn off completely.
- If the injury is near the lacrimal drainage apparatus (i.e. the medial canthus).
- If there are **any** signs of eye damage (including any change in vision).
- If the lid injury is full thickness.

5 If none of these conditions apply then the wound can be closed in the normal way:
- If it is superficial and parallel to the lid margin it can be closed with Steri-strips.
- If it is deeper, gaping or perpendicular to the lid margin it needs to be sutured.
- Deeper tissues can be sutured with 8-0 vicryl while the skin can be closed with 6-0 vicryl so that suture removal is not required.
- If the skin is closed with 7-0 nylon instead, remove the sutures at 1 week.

6 If the injury has involved glass as much of the glass as possible should be removed when exploring the wound (use metal forceps so that the glass can be felt). When all glass appears to have been removed do plain X-rays to check. Again if there is any question of intraocular glass refer immediately.

7 Check tetanus status and give a booster if none has been given in the last 10 years.

8 Generally, systemic antibiotics are not needed as the lids have a very good blood supply. If the injury was particularly dirty, e.g. agricultural or animal, prescribe augmentin 1 tablet tds or erythromycin 500 mg qds for 1 week. Additionally, give metronidazole 500 mg tds to cover anaerobes.

Orbital wall fractures

Whenever there is lid damage it is important to remember that there is the possibility of damage to not only the globe but also the bony orbit. After any trauma the orbital rim should be gently felt for any "steps" that could indicate an underlying fracture. The four walls of the orbit can be damaged in different ways.

Orbital floor fractures (the so-called blow-out fracture)

- The shock waves from blunt trauma to the eye may be conducted to the bony walls of the orbit.
- Two areas of the orbit are particularly prone to damage. The commonest site is the floor of the orbit (i.e. the roof of the maxillary sinus), less commonly the medial wall can be damaged (this usually involves damage to the ethmoid sinuses).
- Because the orbital floor has been damaged part of the orbital contents can herniate into the sinus. This can mean:
  a The globe appears to be "sunken" into the orbit (enophthalmos).
  b The inferior rectus muscle can be tethered in the fracture — the patient is unable to look up.
  c The infraorbital nerve is damaged causing anaesthesia in the area shown in Figure 3.15.
  d Air from the sinus enters the skin (called crepitus or subcutaneous emphysema).
  e Plain X-rays may show the "tear-drop" sign, which is the appearance of the orbital tissue herniating through the fracture.
- Referral of blow-out fractures is to either a maxillofacial or ophthalmic surgeon, although it is important to rule out any associated eye injury at some stage.

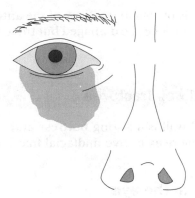

Figure 3.15 The shaded area of skin indicates the extent of anaesthesia after infraorbital nerve damage.

- Most blow-out fractures are asymptomatic and cosmetically acceptable, i.e. do not need surgery.
- Although controversial, if the patient has a history of sinusitis or has a cold at the time of the injury, they should be covered with oral antibiotics, e.g. augmentin 1 tablet tds for 1 week and metronidazole 500 mg tds also for 1 week.

Medial orbital wall fractures

- These rarely cause problems but occasionally patients blow their nose shortly after sustaining the fracture. This forces air into the orbit and subcutaneous tissues causing proptosis and swollen lids, all of which is very dramatic.
- The air absorbs quickly and the patient should be told not to blow their nose for 1 month. Antibiotics are indicated for the same situations as above.
- Very occasionally the medial rectus can become entrapped in the fracture causing double vision when looking **away** from the nose.

Orbital roof fractures

- These are rare but are sometimes missed.
- In any injury that involves a pointed object, such as a garden cane, snooker cue or umbrella tip, penetrating the upper lid may lead to the orbital roof being perforated.

- The orbital roof is of course the floor of the anterior fossa — not only can the frontal lobes be damaged but there is also a high risk of meningitis.

Lateral orbital wall fractures

The lateral orbital wall is a strong buttress and is rarely fractured except as part of more extensive midfacial fractures.

Light damage to the eye

Light in different forms and wavelengths can be harmful to the eye.

Laser pointers

- These low-power laser devices (less than 5 mW) are sometimes purposely shone into someone's eyes either as an intended assault or as a "joke".
- They do not cause ocular damage if looked into momentarily but can cause retinal damage if stared into for several seconds continuously.
- This sort of assault causes considerable distress to the victims and an ophthalmic opinion is usually sought.
- Examination should include visual acuity, corneal examination and a dilated view of the retina, and it is worth bearing in mind that there are often medicolegal overtones.

Solar retinopathy

- Solar retinopathy is caused by infrared rays being focused onto the fovea thereby raising its temperature and causing thermal damage.
- It is most often seen following solar eclipses in which the infrared rays enter the eye in even greater amounts because the pupil dilates in the darkness.
- Occasionally patients are seen who as children played sun-staring games and still have a small central visual scotoma.

- Damage to the vision is variable and although there is no treatment, patients should be referred to an ophthalmologist to assess the degree of damage.

Welding and ultraviolet injuries

- Ultraviolet light in the ultraviolet A (UV-A) and UV-B bands is transmitted by the cornea and absorbed by the lens.
- UV-C is absorbed completely by the cornea and causes epithelial cell loss — the higher the dose the greater the cell loss.
- The three common situations where UV-C corneal burns occur is in welders who have not been using (or who have taken off) their masks, mountain climbers ("snow blindness") and those using sun lamps.
- Typically symptoms come on sometime after UV-C exposure and consist of an intense gritty sensation, watering and some photophobia — when directly questioned the cause is usually obvious.
- Topical anaesthetic, e.g. g. benoxinate stat to both eyes, immediately removes the pain, which is a useful diagnostic clue.
- G. fluorescein 2% and a blue pen-torch or Woods light will show up punctate corneal staining all over both corneas.
- The epithelium heals quickly in 12–24 hours. Until then keep the patient comfortable with Occ. chloramphenicol 2 hourly until the pain eases and then qds for a further 24 hours.
- If the patient is extremely photophobic instill a drop of g. homatropine 1% stat (not atropine as this can dilate the pupil for up to 2 weeks). If this is not available prescribe g. cyclopentolate 1% tds until the pain passes, when it can be stopped.
- Patients should not drive or use machinery until they have stopped the drops and they feel that their vision is back to normal.
- Topical local anaesthetics **cannot** be used as a treatment as they retard epithelial healing.
- It is worth warning the patient that 15–20 minutes after the examination (i.e. as the local anaesthetic wears off) they will feel the pain returning. If the damage is asymmetrical the patient may prefer to have a double pad on the worse eye (see page 143 for instructions on padding). Paracetamol or codeine may also help to relieve the pain until the epithelium heals.

Subtarsal foreign bodies (STFB)

Typical presentation

Presentation is similar to that of a corneal FB, but usually the injuries are of a lower velocity, e.g. windblown.

Because the FB lodges under the upper lid the pain is typically worse on blinking. Typical findings are characteristic scratches in the upper cornea that show up with fluorescein 2% drops and the FB is revealed on everting the lid.

Principles of treatment

1 Precisely define the nature of the injury, i.e. is it low velocity?
2 Check the visual acuity.
3 Look for other foreign bodies or injuries in the eye.

How and what to do

1 Instill a topical anaesthetic into the affected eye, e.g. g. benoxinate.
2 Instill fluorescein 2% drops and illuminate the eye with a blue light (pen-torch, slit-lamp or Woods light).
3 Evert the eyelids:
   – Ask the patient to look down.
   – Take a gentle but firm hold of the upper lid eyelashes.
   – Pull the lid down towards the cheek.
   – Place a cotton bud in the superior half of the upper lid (Figure 3.16a).
   – Pull the lashes forward and upward over the top of the cotton bud (Figure 3.16b).
   – The underside of the upper lid will now be exposed and will remain everted by itself (Figure 3.16c).
4 Wipe the cotton bud along the entire surface of the everted lid to dislodge the STFB.
5 Gently replace the lid.
6 Stat Occ. chloramphenicol.
7 Do not pad unless the patient requests it.

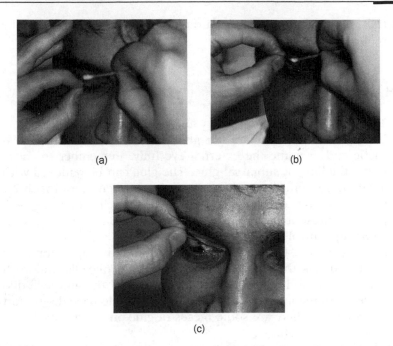

(a)   (b)

(c)

Figure 3.16 (a–c) Technique for everting the eyelid (see text for description).

8 Instruct the patient to return if the eye is still painful 24 hours later.

Superglues and the eye

Typical presentation

Since the advent of extra strong glues a small but steady stream of patients with eye injuries caused by the glue have presented. The diagnosis is usually obvious and may occur as an occupational injury or the glue can be mistaken for eye medications.

Principles of treatment

1 If only the lids are involved the glue can be allowed to dissolve spontaneously.

2 If the patient has glue on the surface of the eye itself it needs to be removed.

How and what to do

1 Take a full history of the injury and its circumstances.
2 If the patient's lashes are not glued shut, instill topical anaes-thetic and examine the external eye fully. Remember to check under the lids for subtarsal glue. The glue can be removed with a cotton bud or a fine pair of forceps. Once removed, instill 2% fluorescein and check for any corneal epithelial damage — if present, prescribe antibiotic ointment for 1 week, e.g. Occ. chloramphenicol qds.
3 If the patient's lashes are glued shut and the eye cannot be examined, ask the patient if they have any ocular discomfort. If they do not, no intervention is necessary and the glue will dis-solve spontaneously after 4 or 5 days. If they do have discomfort this suggests there are some pieces of glue on the eye itself and this cannot be left.
4 Glued lashes are opened by a combination of hot bathing with cotton wool or swabs and cutting the glue or lashes off as necessary.
5 The same principles hold true for children. If the child is in obvious discomfort, the child's lids will need to be opened and any possible glue removed. Depending on the child this may require an EUA.
6 If a child under 7 years of age has had the lids closed for some days, it is prudent, once the lids are opened, to have the child's vision assessed by an orthoptist or optometrist in case of amblyopia.

Trauma to the globe

Typical presentation

The history is usually fairly obvious, i.e. someone or something hit the patient in the eye. Globe injuries can be divided into two main types: (1) when the globe has been perforated (known as a penetrating injury), and (2) when the globe is intact but the con-tents have been damaged (blunt injury).

Full eye examination is vital as signs of injury can be subtle but serious. Imaging of the eye can be useful in certain types of globe injury.

Principles of treatment

1 It is vitally important to take a **detailed** history of the trauma to allow assessment of the forces involved. If the patient is unconscious try to obtain the history from someone who was there at the time.
2 Look for symptoms that suggest serious injury and refer if they are present.
3 Examine the eye carefully looking for possible entry sites for foreign bodies, areas of exposed uveal tissue (indicating globe perforation), or signs of intraocular haemorrhage.
4 Use plain X-rays when the injury is with a radiolucent material.
5 Do not forget to examine for lid and orbital injuries (see page 150).

How and what to do

1 How **exactly** did the injury occur?
   – For various reasons patients may be reluctant to give the full details of the injury, but you need to know what they were doing at the time of the injury, e.g. if they were working were they striking metal onto metal (relatively high risk of IOFB), if they were hit was it with a fist, a ring or a glass?
   – Similarly, if they had an accident at work were they wearing protective glasses — were they the sort of glasses that hug the skin around the eyes or was there space for a FB to get under them?
   – What was the velocity of the object that hit them, e.g. wind-blown objects are extremely unlikely to cause anything more than superficial damage?
   – What was the size of the object that struck them? If it was a small metallic FB think of an IOFB. Squash ball injuries are much more likely to cause eye damage than tennis balls as the latter are bigger than the bony orbit and often hit this rather than the eye itself. Similarly a shuttlecock (the weighted end) often does more damage than a football.

2 What were the symptoms following the injury? Symptoms that may indicate serious ocular injuries are:
   - Sudden reduction in vision that does not recover quickly.
   - Sudden onset of floaters (may indicate vitreous haemorrhage +/− an IOFB).
   - Prolonged photophobia.
3 Approach the eye examination in a systematic way. A drop of topical anaesthetic may make the examination much easier. If the lids are closed by swelling examination is still possible (see page 151). If it is possible that the eye could be ruptured, try not to touch the globe itself as this can cause further damage. Remember to examine both eyes and that in a number of these cases there are going to be legal ramifications.
   - Check the visual acuity and pupillary responses (an RAPD is a very important sign of damage).
   - Check that the eye moves normally by getting the patient to look up/down/left and right.
   - Using a pen-torch, ophthalmoscope or slit-lamp carefully open the lids and look at the conjunctiva and cornea. Look for any areas of exposed uveal (black) tissue protruding from the eye. If you see this refer **immediately** as the globe is perforated. Do not instill antibiotics or tightly pad the eye. Do cover the eye with a single pad (or a plastic shield) attached to the orbital rim rather than pressed onto the eye.
   - If the patient has a subconjunctival haemorrhage he/she will need referral as there could be a perforation underneath.
   - Look at the anterior chamber. Is there obvious haemorrhage in it? This may have settled to form a hyphaema (Figure 3.17).
   - Look at the iris. Is it pulled in one direction (this looks as if the pupil is "pointing" in one direction) — this is highly suspicious of a corneal/scleral perforation (Figure 3.18). Does the pupil move when a light is shone onto it? If not this suggests that the iris has been damaged by the trauma. If the pupil is dilated compared to its fellow this is also suspicious of serious damage (in a **fully conscious** patient this is indicative of ocular rather than cerebral damage)
   - Try to get a red reflex. Whether you dilate the pupil or not depends on your previous findings. In general only do so if no suspicious symptoms or signs are found.
   - If the patient has been using metal on metal or has had a glass injury, plain X-rays can be useful. From a medicolegal point of view they are vital.

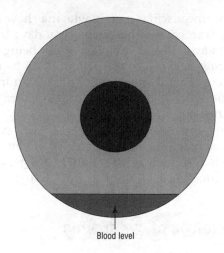

Figure 3.17 Hyphaema.

- If any of the signs or symptoms described above are found, refer the patient to eye casualty that day. Even if there are no definite findings of serious trauma but you are not happy, e.g. high velocity injuries or sharp pointed injuries, then refer.
- Have a very low threshold for referring children with eye injuries.

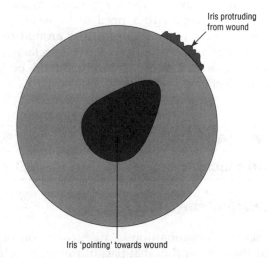

Iris protruding from wound

Iris 'pointing' towards wound

Figure 3.18 A peaked pupil after trauma or surgery is a suspicious sign.

- Similarly, the unconscious patient who may have ocular damage needs to be seen early rather than a few days later when they regain consciousness and complain of not being able to see.
- When referring, make sure the patient is nil by mouth in case they require a general anaesthetic to have an injury repaired. Let the ophthalmologist know past medical history and social circumstances.
- If necessary give systemic analgesia, e.g. paracetamol or codeine phosphate (not aspirin) and an antiemetic.
- Although it is extremely rare for patients to get ocular tetanus, it is a good time to check their tetanus status.

Late complications of eye trauma

It is not unusual for eye injuries to have long-term consequences and it is important to be alert to these:

- Blunt trauma can cause retinal detachment some time after the injury. If the patient complains of increased floaters/flashing lights or a curtain coming over their vision refer at once.
- Months or years after trauma the IOP can increase in the eye. This may well be asymptomatic (like POAG). However, all patients who have had significant blunt trauma should be advised to have an annual IOP check with their optometrist.
- Patients need to be advised about eye safety measures. If they had an industrial accident they need to be wearing regulation eye protection, this is usually close fitting around the eyes, i.e. elasticated goggles rather than protective spectacles. Similarly, patients who have had sports injuries should be advised to wear specially designed eye protectors.

Chronic visual loss

Age related macular degeneration (ARMD or AMD)

Typical presentation

Age related macular degeneration is a degeneration of the retina that occurs at the macula (i.e. that part of the retina with the best vision) in patients over the age of 50. Although there are two main types of ARMD — the "dry" and "wet" type — the vast majority of patients have the dry type for which there is no proven treatment.

The wet or exudative type is so called because a leash of new vessels grows into the macula. In a small number of patients these vessels can be closed off with laser treatment, although the likelihood of recurrence is high.

Patients with dry ARMD tend to have a gradual loss of vision over months and years, typically complaining of difficulty with reading or fine work and difficulty in distinguishing faces. Visual acuity is variable, some patients being as good as 6/9 or 6/12, whilst others can decline to 6/60 or HMS. As only the central vision is affected, the patients never lose vision completely.

Patients with the wet type of ARMD tend to present suddenly with distortion of vision (caused by a lacy network of new vessels physically distorting the macula) complaining that straight lines such as door or window frames have become wobbly. If the vessels bleed, the central vision declines suddenly.

Principles of treatment

1 Dry ARMD is not an urgent condition. Many patients have no symptoms from it and do not require hospital referral. However, if they are symptomatic, referral can have advantages for the patient.
2 Wet ARMD needs immediate referral — if treatment is to be effective it must be performed as early as possible. Even delaying for 24 hours can affect the eventual outcome as the neovascular membrane (NVM) can grow rapidly.
3 ARMD is a bilateral disease and patients need to be warned of the risk to the fellow eye — especially in those with wet ARMD.

How and what to do

1 **Dry ARMD:**
   - Often picked up by an optometrist during an eye test.
   - Check the distance and reading vision.
   - If you check the visual fields they will be normal, but the patient may lose the fixation target (unless it is a large target) when it approaches central vision.

- ARMD does **not** cause an afferent pupillary defect — pupil reactions would be expected to be normal.
- Dilate the pupils and look at the macula — during ophthalmoscopy, if the patient is asked to look straight into your light, you will then be looking straight at the macula (see page 48).
- The macula may have a number of features including small white dots (drusen), atrophic/grey areas, or prominent (choroidal) vessels. The difference between the area of macular degeneration and the normal surrounding retina is usually fairly obvious.
- If the patient has no visual complaints (in fact only 10% of those with dry ARMD report visual problems) they do not need specialist referral. They should be advised to have an eye test every year and warned of the symptoms of distortion (see below).
- If they have visual problems associated with their ARMD refer them routinely to ophthalmic outpatients' department. Here they will have a full ocular examination (it is not unusual in this age group for cataract to coexist with ARMD) and assessment of need for magnifying devices (called low visual aids or LVAs). If the vision is very poor the patient may be eligible for blind or partial sight registration — this can only be done by a consultant ophthalmologist (for the criteria and benefits of registration see pages 200–202).
- One of the most important things to do for patients with ARMD is to assure them that although they have lost some of their central reading vision they will never lose their peripheral (which is what they navigate with) vision. This is often of great comfort to the sufferers.

2 Wet (exudative) AMD:
- The onset of this type of ARMD is sudden (days). It may occur in patients known to have ARMD or it may be the first presentation.
- The cardinal symptom is **distortion of straight lines** — anyone with sudden onset of distortion needs immediate referral to eye casualty. In the early stages vision may be near normal but if the patient is asked to close the unaffected eye and look at a window or door frame they will describe an area where the vertical line is distorted. Similarly if they look at a page of text they will describe an area where the print is bent or distorted (for further explanation of examining for distortion see pages 29–31).

- Dilating the pupils may reveal a raised area around the macula, often with overlying or surrounding haemorrhage. Whatever the examination findings refer the patient by telephone.
- In eye casualty, the patient will undergo fluorescein angiography. Fluorescein is injected intravenously and is carried by the circulation to the choroid where it delineates the extent of the new vessels. The picture this gives is used to guide the laser treatment. The purpose of the laser is to seal off the new vessels and prevent them proliferating without damaging more retina
- Although laser treatment has been shown to be effective, only certain types of NVM can be treated and the recurrence rate is very high.
- If a patient has an NVM in one eye they have a high risk (roughly 10% per year) of having one in the fellow eye. The most sensitive indicator of an NVM forming is the onset of distortion, so that patients are advised to check daily for it. This is done using a window or door frame or using a special chart with a central fixation target and horizontal and vertical lines (called an Amsler chart, see page 30).
- Whatever the method used to detect it, sudden distortion requires immediate attendance at eye casualty.

Cataract

Typical presentation

Patients usually complain of a gradual loss of vision in one or both eyes. If they drive they complain particularly of glare from headlights at night. They may have already consulted their optometrist.

Principles of treatment

1 How disabled is the patient by the cataract?
2 Can the vision be improved by refraction?
3 Only refer the patient if they would actually want to have surgery.
4 If after cataract extraction a patient feels like "the cataract is coming back" they may have posterior capsule opacification.

How and what to do

1 To obtain a measure of how disabled the patient is by their cataract, enquire into difficulties with their work, hobbies, or driving. Do they have any other disabilities? Do they live alone?

2 Check the visual acuity both distance and near, see if it improves with a pinhole (this may indicate that the vision is partially correctable by refraction; see page 26).

3 Check for an afferent pupillary defect; a cataract does **not** cause an afferent pupillary defect and if present other pathology must be suspected.

4 Check for a red reflex using a direct ophthalmoscope shone at the eye from arm's length in a dark room (see Figure 2.10, page 49). A red/orange glow is reflected back from the fundus if the optical media are clear. If a lens opacity is present it will block the light and will be seen as dark against the red reflex. If the lens is completely opacified, no red reflex at all will be seen.

5 If you have dilating drops available, e.g. tropicamide 1% or cyclopentolate 0.5–1%, dilate the pupil. This will allow an easier view of the red reflex and posterior pole. For guidelines on dilating see pages 62–63.

6 If the patient has not had a sight test recently it is usually worth referring them to an optometrist.

7 If the optometrist cannot correct the vision and the patient is prepared to undergo surgery then refer to an ophthalmologist routinely. If there are visual or social factors for an earlier appointment let the ophthalmologist know.

8 What you need to tell the patient if they have been referred:
   - That they have been referred for **consideration** of cataract surgery.
   - The name of the consultant they have been referred to.
   - The operation is usually done under local anaesthetic as a day case, but general anesthesia is available. It is now very rare not to insert an intraocular lens at the time of surgery.
   - Although the surgery is safe and highly effective, around 10% of patients will have no improvement in visual acuity following surgery. One per cent will require further surgery and around 1/1000 patients will lose vision.
   - You should warn them that they will probably have to change their glasses' prescription after cataract surgery.

Posterior capsule opacification ("secondary cataract")

- The intraocular implant is usually placed on the posterior capsule of the lens during surgery (the anterior capsule being removed at the time of surgery).
- Over time this capsule can itself opacify and it can appear to the patient that the cataract has returned.
- This may be seen as a darkening of the red reflex again.
- The treatment of this is relatively simple (although not, of course, without its own potential complications) and involves a quick outpatient laser ablation of the thickened capsule.

Diabetes and the eye

As with the rest of the body, diabetes can have a wide range of different complications in the eye. The main ones encountered in practice are discussed below. Undoubtedly the most common ocular complication is diabetic retinopathy — and probably the most important as it is sight threatening — but it can be avoided by early detection and treatment.

Lids

- Styes.
- Lid cellulitis and other bacterial infections are more common in diabetics.

Lens

- Diabetics have a higher prevalence of cataract and it tends to develop at a younger age.
- Occasionally teenage diabetics can present with poor diabetic control and almost white cataracts. These can sometimes be completely reversed simply by normalising the blood sugar.
- Diabetics can undergo symptomatic changes in vision because of variations in blood sugar levels. The changes are due to variations

in lens thickness because of the high sugar. This stabilises when blood sugar is more tightly controlled.

Extraocular muscles

- Diabetics are prone to microvascular disease and if one of the blood vessels supplying one of the extraocular muscles is blocked the muscle will fail to work. Clinically this presents as sudden onset of double vision and is discussed on page 105. Usually these palsies resolve in around 6 weeks.
- Acute IIIrd nerve palsies occurring secondary to diabetic microvascular disease are classically differentiated from IIIrd nerve palsies caused by posterior communicating artery aneurysms because the latter have pupillary (dilated) involvement. However, although this rule is generally true, posterior communicating artery aneurysms **can** occur without pupil involvement and all patients with acute IIIrd nerve palsies should be referred to an ophthalmologist or neurologist urgently.

Diabetic retinopathy

- Diabetic retinopathy can sometimes be the presenting feature of diabetes, although this is increasingly rare.
- More often the retinopathy is picked up via screening.
- The most important risk factor for the development of diabetic retinopathy is how long the patient has been diabetic. More than 60% of diabetics develop retinopathy after 15 years of diabetes.
- In juvenile diabetes mellitus, proliferative diabetic retinopathy (PDR) is uncommon in patients younger than 20 years and almost unheard of in patients younger than 16 years.
- The risk of losing vision from diabetic retinopathy increases with the duration of the diabetes.
- Visual loss occurs because of maculopathy or proliferative diabetic retinopathy — early diagnosis and treatment (laser) can prevent visual loss from these.
- Newly diagnosed diabetics need dilated fundoscopy, if they have no background retinopathy they need a yearly check.
- This can be carried out by an optometrist, GP, or diabetologist. It is now suggested that it is done by "suitably trained and experienced practitioners".

If possible screening should:

a Ask about any recent changes in vision.

b Measure the best visual acuity.

c Dilate the pupil with tropicamide 1% to both eyes (for instructions for dilating the pupil see pages 62–63).

d Look for lens opacities.

e Examine the optic nerve, macula, and the blood vessels.

- An alternative to this screening examination, popular in some areas, is taking retinal photographs and then either a diabetologist or ophthalmologist examines them for abnormalities. This is much cheaper but less sensitive.
- It is important to remember that other factors contribute to worsening of diabetic retinopathy:

a poor diabetic control

b systemic hypertension

c hyperlipidaemia

d smoking

e anaemia

f renal disease.

Drugs and the eye

Drug abuse and the eye

It is important to be aware that drug abuse (both legal and illegal) can have specific effects on the eye, some of which can be improved with treatment.

Tobacco/alcohol amblyopia

- This was initially thought to be due to the toxic effects of nicotine and alcohol on the optic nerve.
- It now appears to be due to vitamin B deficiency (probably B_{12} and thiamine), i.e. it has more to do with lifestyle and nutrition rather than a direct toxic effect.
- Anyone who may be at risk of malnutrition and who complains of rapidly failing vision should be referred to an ophthalmologist urgently to assess for a vitamin deficiency related optic neuropathy, as the loss is potentially reversible with treatment.

Methanol ingestion

- Can occur accidentally with "home-made" alcohol or purposely in alcoholics.
- Even in small amounts can cause blindness.
- Symptoms of decreased visual acuity appear at 24–48 hours after ingestion and there is often optic disc swelling.
- Emergency medical referral is mandatory as the mortality rate is very high.
- Treatment is with sodium bicarbonate and ethanol.
- If patients do not show improvement in visual acuity within 1 week it is unlikely it will improve much.

Intravenous drug abuse

- Risk of septic emboli leading to endophthalmitis (intraocular infection).
- Infection often with atypical organisms such as *Candida, Aspergillus, Bacillus cereus*.
- IV drug abusers with reduction in vision and a red eye should be referred to an ophthalmologist the same day.
- IV drug abusers may also get retinal emboli from odd sources such as talcum powder that has been injected intravenously.
- These patients present with a sudden, painless decrease in vision.

General anaesthesia and the eye

The various components of general anaesthetics can have ocular complications. Conversely there are a number of drugs and techniques used in ophthalmology which need to be taken into consideration during anaesthesia.

Ocular complications caused by anaesthetists

Intraocular pressure

- Most general anaesthetics lower the IOP therefore producing false readings. This is particularly important in children undergoing EUA and many paediatric ophthalmologists prefer ketamine.

- Some anaesthetics, such as succinylcholine, actually increase IOP, probably by increasing extraocular muscle tone. Further, intubation, laryngeal spasm, retching and vomiting dramatically increase the IOP. Although this is harmless for short periods it can be disastrous if the globe is open. Succinylcholine is avoided for anaesthesia for operations to repair open eye injuries.
- Dilation or constriction of the pupil can occur under general anaesthesia. Constriction may be a problem during cataract or retinal surgery. Pupil dilation can put susceptible patients into closed angle glaucoma — beware the patient who awakens from general anaesthesia with a red eye.

The cornea

The cornea is vulnerable to damage during (non-ophthalmic) general anaesthesia because:
- Lid closure is abnormal, this means the cornea can dry out during the procedure. This is avoided by taping the lids shut.
- The protective lid reflex is lost, so protection against corneal abrasion is lost.
- The corneal touch reflex itself is lost in deep anaesthesia, increasing the likelihood of damage.
- Some agents (e.g. nitrous oxide, halothane) reduce tear production which also increases the possibility of corneal damage.
- The postoperative patient with a red eye caused by closed angle glaucoma is unavoidable, whereas when the red eye is because of a corneal abrasion it is entirely avoidable.

Others

- Inadvertent spillage of alcohol-based skin prepping solutions around the eye can cause corneal burns.
- Succinylcholine should not be used when forced duction testing (an examination technique that involves the examiner forcibly moving the eye around in an attempt to judge if any of the eye muscles are tethered) is being contemplated, as it causes muscle contraction.
- When intraocular gas is used to tamponade retinal holes, nitrous oxide cannot be used as it will expand the gas inside the eye.

General anaesthetic complications caused by ophthalmologists

General anaesthesia can itself be affected by drugs used on the eye or manoeuvres used during ophthalmic surgery:

• Manipulation of the extraocular muscles during anaesthesia can produce a very profound bradycardia. It is important for this reflex to be blunted with IV atropine.

• If mannitol is used to reduce IOP during intraocular surgery, the incidence of pulmonary oedema is increased as is the postoperative incidence of urinary retention.

• Cocaine-soaked nasal packs sometimes used prior to lacrimal surgery can be absorbed systemically causing tachycardia, arrhythmias and an increase in blood pressure.

• Phenylephrine, used to dilate the pupil, can also cause tachycardia and hypertension during anaesthesia.

• Acetylcholine (Miochol or Miostat) is sometimes used intraocularly to constrict the pupil. It can cause hypotension and bradycardia during and shortly after GA (rare).

Hydroxychloroquine, chloroquine and the eye

Typical presentation

Hydroxychloroquine and chloroquine can cause irreversible loss of vision due to retinal toxicity. They are usually used in the treatment of rheumatoid arthritis, systemic lupus erythromatosis or cutaneous lupus. The advice given below is based on the Royal College of Ophthalmologists' Guidelines for Screening published in 1998.

How and what to do

1 It is recommended that first line treatment is with hydroxychloroquine as it is much less toxic than chloroquine, the latter only being used if other agents have failed. Toxicity is dependent on the cumulative dose taken. For chloroquine there is inadequate data to give a maximum safe dose. However it has been found that for hydroxychloroquine, ocular toxicity is very rare for

doses below 6.5 mg/kg/day, although after 6 years of treatment it becomes more common.

2 Toxicity may be reversible (corneal epithelial changes or loss of foveal light reflex) or irreversible (the so-called "Bulls-eye" maculopathy appearance). Patients do not usually complain of any visual symptoms until the bulls-eye stage is reached.

3 Screening programmes and baseline examinations by ophthalmologists are not justified.

4 Monitoring is performed by the doctor who initiates the treatment. Current guidelines suggest:

Before starting on treatment:
- Check renal and liver function.
- Ask if there are any visual problems currently — if present refer patient to their optometrist.
- Check near visual acuity (see pages 28–29, or obtain the guidelines from the Royal College of Ophthalmologists which contains appropriate test types). Use the patient's reading glasses if he/she uses them normally.
- Warn the patient to contact you immediately if he/she experiences any alteration in their vision.

Ongoing evaluation:
- The visual checks are performed yearly — unless the patient has visual symptoms in between visits.
- At these checks ask about visual symptoms.
- Recheck acuity.

5 Refer to an ophthalmologist if:
- Eye disease is detected at baseline assessment that cannot be improved by the optometrist.
- The patient develops symptoms or signs of visual alteration.
- A child is being treated.

Steroids and the eye

Topical and systemic corticosteroids are, of course, a vital treatment of modern ophthalmology. However, steroids can have serious ocular side effects, some of which are potentially blinding.

Indications for topical steroids

Topical steroids are commonly used by ophthalmologists to treat a range of inflammatory conditions. Some examples include acute anterior uveitis, scleritis, severe atopy, non-infectious keratitis, and severe lid margin disease. They are also used after intraocular surgery to reduce the inflammatory response, especially after cataract extraction or trabeculectomy.

Typical dosage regimes can vary from hourly in severe inflammations to alternate days when there is a need for slow withdrawal. Topical ocular steroids vary in their potency (and to some extent their side effects):

Fluromethalone
Prednisolone 0.3%
Prednisolone 0.5%
Dexamethasone 0.1%
Prednisolone Forte

Increasingly potent

Ocular side effects of topical steroids

Any type of steroid can cause ocular side effects if taken for a sufficient amount of time in susceptible patients. Oral, inhaled and topical steroid (especially on the face) have all been reported to produce these ocular complications and patients on long-term steroids should be advised to see their optometrist for regular examinations.

However, topical ocular steroids are far more likely to cause ocular side effects than do other forms and should be used **only** if the patient has access to an ophthalmically trained practitioner with the appropriate specialised equipment.

The potential complications of steroids are:

- cataract formation
- herpes simplex keratitis
- raising of IOP and subsequent glaucoma
- bacterial keratitis
- thinning of the cornea.

Systemic effects of eye medications

The systemic effects of ocular medications can easily be overlooked. It is important to remember that a substantial proportion of eye drops will drain into the highly vascular nasolacrimal duct. The subsequent absorption passes into the systemic circulation, i.e. there is no first-pass metabolism from the liver.

For many eye drops this is not important as their systemic effects are minimal but certain eye medications can have profound systemic effects. Ointments hold the active drug in the conjunctiva and are associated with a lower incidence of systemic side effects. Reduction of systemic absorption can also occur if patients close their eyes for 5 minutes after instillation or press at the medial canthus for around the same length of time The potential for side effects is very much greater in children.

Topical beta-blockers

Use

Highly effective lowering of intraocular pressure.

Examples

Timolol (Timoptol), laevobunolol (Betagan), betaxolol (Betoptic).

Possible side effects

Topical beta-blockers can cause exactly the same side effects as oral (one drop of 0.5% g. timolol is the equivalent of a 10 mg oral dose). This means that a full medical history is taken prior to initiating treatment and if side effects develop the drop is changed. Potential side effects are:

- *Respiratory*:
  - Contraindicated in asthmatics and COAD.
  - Can subtly reduce exercise tolerance in the elderly. (Betaxalol is cardioselective but is still contraindicated in airways disease).
- *Cardiac*:
  - Bradycardia.
  - Falls and blackouts.
- *Neurological*:
  - Stroke.
  - Nightmares.
  - Depression.

- *Other*:
  - Impotence.

Alpha-agonists

Use

Lower IOP.

Examples

Brimonidine (Alphagan), dipivefrine (Propine), apraclonidine (Iopidine).

Possible side effects

Contraindicated in severe cardiovascular disease. Have the potential for causing arrhythmias, raising BP, and worsening of angina. Non-specific lethargy/depression.

Carbonic anhydrase inhibitors

Use

Lower IOP.

Examples

- Systemic: acetazolamide (Diamox).
- Topical: dorzolamide (Trusopt).

Possible side effects

Acetazolamide is notorious for causing a myriad of systemic side effects including acid/base imbalance, renal stones, tingling of the fingers, malaise and anorexia, bone-marrow suppression, Stevens–Johnson syndrome, and hypokalaemia (usually only if on other diuretics also). Acetazolamide continues to be used so widely because it is so effective at reducing the IOP; however, long-term use is avoided if at all possible as is use in children.

Dorzolamide is a topical carbonic anhydrase inhibitor and has a much lower incidence of systemic side effects (as well as a lower IOP lowering effect). It is important to remember that it has the potential for the same side effects as its systemic counterpart.

Miotics

Uses

Constrict the pupil, lower, IOP.

Examples

Pilocarpine, carbachol.

Possible side effects

These drugs are parasympathomimetics and, although rare, anticholinergic side effects such as bradycardia, confusion, abdominal cramp, and urinary retention can occur. These side effects are more likely in very elderly patients.

Phenylephrine

Use

Pupil dilation (in combination with cyclopentolate or tropicamide).

Examples

Phenylephrine 2.5% or 10%.

Possible side effects

Although not consistent, there have been a number of reports of problems with topical phenylephrine such as arrhythmias and hypertension — usually associated with the 10% concentration. Generally it is best avoided in children, the elderly and those with cardiovascular disease, but if it is necessary to get maximal pupil dilation use 2.5% and repeat as minimally as possible.

Antimuscarinics

Uses

Pupil dilation, paralysis of accommodation (for refraction in children).

Examples

Atropine, cyclopentolate, tropicamide.

Possible side effects

Antimuscarinics can cause bradycardia, nausea and vomiting, dizziness, and urinary retention. In adults this is rarely a problem but, again, in children and the elderly side effects can occur. In these groups, pupil dilation is most safely achieved with g. tropicamide 0.5%. If accommodative paralysis is required g. cyclopentolate 0.5% or 1% is needed. Sometimes it is difficult to dilate children with very dark irises and in this situation the child may be sent home with atropine 1% ointment (to reduce systemic absorption) to be used for 2–3 days prior to the next appointment. It is important, if this is done, that the parents are informed of the symptoms and signs of atropine toxicity and told to stop the treatment immediately and consult a medical practitioner.

G. atropine or g. cyclopentolate are used in the treatment of acute anterior uveitis to maintain pupil dilation and there is a small risk of systemic toxicity.

Topical steroids

Use

Suppression of ocular inflammation.

Examples

Dexamethasone (Maxidex), prednisolone (Predsol).

Possible side effects

In some ocular conditions fortified topical steroids are given in large amounts, e.g. hourly, however reports of clinically significant side effects are very rare — perhaps because intensive treatment is only for a short duration. Although there are no data, it is prudent to keep topical steroids to a minimum in pregnant women and very young children.

Topical antibiotics

Use

Superficial ocular infections.

Examples

Chloramphenicol, gentamicin, fucidic acid, tetracycline.

Possible side effects

Again in certain ocular infections fortified antibiotics are given frequently but reports of systemic toxicity are extremely rare. Again in children and pregnant women it may be best to avoid frequent gentamicin.

There have been a number of reports of bone-marrow suppression in patients who were taking topical chloramphenicol. These reactions seem to be idiosyncratic and ophthalmologists continue to use it as a first line treatment. For peace of mind it is better to use ointment rather than drops, avoid in very young children, and do not use for longer than is necessary.

With most of these medications the prescription is initiated by an ophthalmologist. However if you suspect that a patient is having side effects from their ocular medications it is important to contact the appropriate consultant or a pharmacist experienced in ophthalmic drugs and their side effects. Once again, it is important to remember that the drugs in eye drops have the potential to cause serious systemic side effects.

Miscellaneous

Contact lens problems

Typical presentation

The vast majority of people who wear contact lenses have no

problems at all. Of those that do, most problems are trivial and self limiting. However there is a small risk that contact lenses, especially if they are worn for long periods or if hygiene instructions are not followed, can give rise to sight-threatening infections.

Presenting symptoms range from itch if patients become allergic to their lens cleaning solutions to pain, photophobia, and decreased vision of infective keratitis.

Principles of treatment

1 Contact lens (CL) wearers can present with a number of different symptoms. Separate the sight-threatening problems from the non-sight-threatening, with the former going to see an ophthalmologist and the latter going to see their contact lens practitioner (CLP).
2 If a CL wearer has a red or sticky eye they should **stop wearing their lenses** until it has settled.
3 If a CL wearer has any epithelial loss/disturbance they need to have antibiotic cover until it has healed.
4 Many eye drops cannot be used when CL are in — always check with the patient whether they are wearing lenses and with the manufacturer's instructions on the medications.
5 Any CL wearer with pain, photophobia or decreased vision (i.e. symptoms of keratitis) needs immediate ophthalmic referral.

How and what to do

Contact lenses are of three main types: hard, soft and gas permeable (which are hard but have holes in them to increase oxygen supply to the cornea). To some extent complications are related to the type of lens worn. Common CL-related problems that present are:

1 Wearing lenses for too many hours (overwear).
2 Allergy to CL solutions.
3 Bacterial keratitis.
4 Acanthamoeba keratitis.
5 CL stuck.
6 CL-induced abrasions.
7 Poor lens hygiene.

1 When a CL patient presents with discomfort, redness or pain it is important to take a detailed history, as this often is the clue to the underlying problem:
   - How many hours a day does the patient wear their lenses?
   - Overwear is rarely a problem with hard or gas permeable lenses as it is too uncomfortable to keep them in for a long period.
   - Soft lenses are much more comfortable and can be worn for long stretches of time.
   - If a patient is wearing the lenses for more than 12 hours a day and is getting discomfort, the patient should be advised to remove the lenses and consult his/her CLP.
   - If there is corneal staining due to the overwear, cover the patient with antibiotics, e.g. g. chloramphenicol qds for 1 week. They should not see their CLP until they have stopped the drops.

2 If the predominant symptom is itch:
   - The patient may have become sensitive to some of the cleaning solutions.
   - The simplest thing to do is to recommend taking a break from the CL for a couple of weeks and to see if there is an improvement. After this period the patient should see their CLP.
   - If leaving out the lenses removes the itch the patient can try hypoallergenic CL solutions.
   - Allergic conjunctivitis in CL wearers is not always the fault of the lens and may simply be an exacerbation of pre-existing allergic eye disease.
   - If lens removal or hypoallergenic solutions do not help try g. opticrom tds for 1 month. If there is no relief refer routinely to an ophthalmologist.

3 Bacterial keratitis:
   - Presents with a very painful, photophobic eye with reduced visual acuity and a visible white patch on the cornea representing the infected area (see Figure 3.4, page 110).
   - The usual cause is extended wear (soft) CL and it is now stipulated that CLs should not be worn overnight.
   - Any patient who appears to have or is developing signs of a keratitis (pain, photophobia, decreased vision) needs to be referred immediately to an ophthalmologist.
   - The patient should be instructed to take their CLs, their solutions and case to the hospital with them.

4 Acanthamoeba keratitis:
   - A rare but potentially devastating amoebic infection of the cornea. It is a very rare infection but more common in CL wearers.

- The main risk factor is cleaning the CL with tap water.
- Signs of acanthamoeba include intense pain in the eye early in the disease when the cornea may be clear.
- Later a dendritic-like corneal epithelial loss can be seen with 2% fluorescein (**Note:** never put fluorescein into an eye with a CL in as it will stain the lens.)
- Any CL wearer with a unilateral red eye who admits to washing their lenses in tap water should be discussed with an ophthalmologist.

5 Sometimes patients present because they have a CL stuck either on the cornea or under the upper lid:
- Anaesthetise the eye with minims of g. benoxinate or g. amethocaine.
- If the CL is stuck on the cornea locate it using a slit-lamp or good illumination with magnification.
- Place your thumb and index finger either side of the lens and slowly move them towards each other, this should "pinch" the lens in the middle and it can be lifted off.
- If the lens has got stuck under the upper lid, evert the lid (see pages 156–157), run a cotton bud along the entire length of the lid and this should bring the lens with it.
- Unfortunately, lost CL have a habit of lodging high up in the superior fornix — either evert once and run a cotton bud **under** the everted lid or repeat the everting so that the lid is double-everted (difficult) and the superior fornix is exposed.
- Even after removal it is not uncommon for the patient to still have foreign body symptoms — this is probably due to the manipulation and it soon passes.
- If you cannot find a CL reassure the patient and asked the patient to return the following morning if the discomfort is still felt.
- If the patient does return have a look again then, if you are unable to find the CL, refer the patient to eye casualty.

6 If the patient complains of sudden, severe pain when they were inserting or removing their CL then they probably have a CL-induced abrasion of the cornea:
- This can be confirmed (after the lens is removed) by instilling 2% fluorescein and using a blue light.
- Do **not** pad the eye but prescribe Occ. chloramphenicol 2 hourly for 24 hours. If the patient is very photophobic also prescribe g. cylopentolate 1% tds for 48 hours.
- The patient should be warned to return immediately if the pain

worsens or the vision drops as there is a higher risk of bacterial keratitis.

- Review the patient the next day. If the patient is symptomatically improved and the abrasion is smaller, reduce the Occ. chloramphenicol to qds and continue it for a further week.
- At the end of the treatment the patient should be instructed to see their CLP for a lens check before putting their lenses in again.
- Poor lens cleaning can cause chronic irritation due to a build up of debris. The patient needs to remove the lenses and attend their CLP.
- Occasionally patients present who have not fully removed the hydrogen peroxide cleaner from the lens. This tends to be immediately painful. Treatment is to remove the lens, irrigate the eye (see pages 136–137), and prescribe chloramphenicol ointment until the epithelium heals.

Dizziness

Typical presentation

It is not rare for a patient with dizziness to present to the doctor querying whether "their eyes could be the problem". However, true dizziness is **never** a visual problem.

How and what to do

1 Take a careful history looking for both ocular and ENT symptoms.
2 If the patient complains of the **room spinning around** then this is true dizziness (i.e. vertigo) and needs referral to an ENT surgeon.
3 If the patient is complaining of falling due to poor vision then full ophthalmic assessment is required. The minimum required is visual acuity, confrontation fields, pupil responses and fundoscopy. Further referral depends on the findings.
4 Of course true dizziness and eye disease can coexist and any sort of visual problem will greatly exacerbate any balance problems the patient is experiencing.
5 Check lying and standing blood pressure and FBC.

Glaucoma referral from optometrist

Typical presentation

The patient will usually be referred following a routine sight test and have a GOS 18 form containing the optometrist's findings (see page 18). The optometrist usually suspects primary open angle glaucoma (POAG), but occasionally closed angle is suspected, patients are therefore usually asymptomatic.

How and what to do

1 The patient will need onward referral.
2 If the optometrist suspects POAG then send the GOS 18 form with any extra information required to the eye outpatients department.
3 If there is any suspicion of closed angle glaucoma from either the form or the patient's symptoms (episodes of eye pain and haloes/rainbows around lights), then discuss immediately with the on-call ophthalmologist.
4 Give past medical and drug history, either on the GOS 18 form or attached to it.
5 Explain to the patient:
   - Glaucoma is a disease usually caused by raised pressure in the eye resulting in damage to the nerve at the back of the eye.
   - It usually progresses slowly and can often be effectively treated just with drops, although these need to be taken life long.
   - They have been referred to an eye specialist, but that they do not need to be seen urgently. However, if an appointment date has not been received within 6 weeks they should contact you again.

HIV and the eye

Typical presentation

Most patients presenting with eye manifestations of AIDS are known to be HIV positive, although the eye complications can sometimes be the first clue to the diagnosis. AIDS can affect

Table 3.1 The main ocular complications of AIDS

Complication	Finding
Herpes zoster ophthalmicus	Vesicular lesions and ocular involvement, both anterior and posterior segment. Often involves more than one dermatome
Kaposi's sarcoma	Bright red subconjunctival lesion usually in inferior conjunctiva
CMV retinopathy	A mixture of haemorrhagic and white lesions in the retina
AIDS retinopathy	Cotton-wool spots, flame-shaped and dot haemorrhages, Roth's spots
Toxoplasmosis	Yellow white retinochoroidal lesion, single or multiple, vitritis may be prominent, usually no retinal haemorrhages
Candida retinitis	Yellow white fluffy lesions, usually multiple, vitritis and vitreous abscess present, retinal haemorrhages
Pneumocystis carinii	Multiple yellow choroidal lesions, no vascular involvement or vitritis
Neuro-ophthalmic involvement	Cranial nerve palsies, optic neuritis

almost any part of the eye. Typically patients present with opportunistic infections such as herpes zoster ophthalmicus (HZO) or cytomegalovirus (CMV) retinitis. Some of the main manifestations are listed in Table 3.1.

Principles of treatment

Patients can lose vision permanently if not treated urgently and therefore a low threshold for referral is important.

How and what to do

1 The more minor complications of ocular AIDS, e.g. blepharitis, can be treated as they would normally (see relevant topics).
2 If an HIV positive patient has visual symptoms they need a full ophthalmic examination, including dilated fundoscopy. Whatever the findings, discuss with the on-call ophthalmologist.

3 If the patient has ocular features of AIDS but is **not** known to be HIV positive:
   – If the presenting feature is non-vision threatening, e.g. Kaposi's sarcoma of the conjunctiva, then refer the patient urgently to an infectious disease specialist.
   – If there is a vision-threatening problem then refer the patient immediately to an eye clinic.
4 The range of ocular complications of HIV is large. Table 3.1 indicates some of the more common and important ones and the typical findings associated with them.

Imaging and the eye

Plain X-rays in ophthalmology

Plain X-rays are not often used in modern ophthalmology but there are some situations in which they are useful:

Locating metallic intraocular foreign bodies (IOFBs)

• Anyone who gives a history of something going into their eye whilst using metal on metal needs to have orbital X-rays.
• The commonest scenario is when using a hammer and chisel. The metal fragment is small, sharp and travelling at high velocity — ideal circumstances for entering the eye.
• Other scenarios include drilling metal or grinding, although the latter rarely seems to cause ocular penetration.
• Even if a superficial FB is found, all patients with metal on metal eye injuries need orbital (AP and lateral) X-rays for evidence of an IOFB.
• The possibility of missing a small fragment with an X-ray is quite high. If there is anything suspicions in the history, such as a change in vision or a definite history of an FB flying into the eye but none can be located, referral to eye casualty for dilated fundoscopy is mandatory.

Glass injuries

• Glass with high lead content will sometimes show up on plain X-rays and can be useful when someone has sustained an ocular or peri-orbital glass injury.

- It does not however replace a careful examination and if necessary surgical exploration.

Blow-out fractures

- Fractures of the orbital floor (i.e. the roof of the maxillary sinus) with prolapse of the part of the orbital contents are known as a blow-out fracture.
- They can lead to diplopia and/or poor cosmesis and may need surgical exploration and repair.
- In the acute situation, plain facial X-rays are useful to confirm the clinical impression of a blow-out fracture.
- A fracture line may be seen along the orbital rim and sometimes a hypodense shadow beneath this (the so-called teardrop sign), which represents herniation of orbital tissue into the sinus and is strongly suggestive of a blow-out fracture.
- If surgical intervention is contemplated, a CT scan is required for more precise location of the fracture.

CT scanning in ophthalmology

CT scanning is as ubiquitous in ophthalmology as in other branches of medicine. As CT scanning is most useful for imaging bony structures, the commonest indications are for structures of the orbit and retro-orbit.

Orbital walls

- Blow-out fractures can be localised and delineated by CT scanning.
- Fractures of the medial orbital wall (lamina papyracea) are best identified by CT.

Optic canal

- Fractures of the optic canal can occur after severe head injury — they are more common when the injury is to the forehead and are usually associated with loss of consciousness.
- If the optic nerve itself is damaged any visual loss may not be recognised until the patient regains consciousness.
- CT scanning of the optic canal can allow identification of the fracture in the unconscious patient and treatment can be instituted.

- The most important way of diagnosing optic canal fracture is to have a high index of suspicion and to convey this to the radiologist so that appropriate scans can be ordered.

Orbital contents

- A number of orbital pathologies can be identified with CT, such as tumours, inflammation, or infiltration.
- It is important to specify to the radiologist that orbital pathology is suspected so that 4-mm sections can be performed.

Pituitary fossa

- This is combined with serum prolactin levels, the investigation of choice in patients with bitemporal visual field loss to exclude pituitary pathology.
- Again it is important to specify to the radiologist the possibility of pituitary pathology.

MRI and ophthalmology

- MRI is extremely valuable for soft-tissue abnormalities including those of the orbital contents and brain.
- Precise imaging of orbital pathology, e.g. extent of tumour spread, can be obtained, as well as precise location of neurophthalmic lesions, e.g. cranial nerve or optic pathway lesions.
- MRI can be so precise that even some ocular injuries/abnormalities can be imaged.
- However, because of the strong magnets involved, if a metallic IOFB is suspected, MRI should not be used as it may move the FB within the eye.
- Similarly, patients who have had cranial aneurysms clipped should not undergo MRI as there is a risk, with the older types, of moving the clip.

Ultrasonography in ophthalmology

- This is undoubtedly the commonest form of imaging used in ophthalmology and is used to measure the eye and to image ocular structures obscured by any media opacities.

- Specifically designed ophthalmic ultrasound probes are used and the technique does require some experience. There are two types of ophthalmic ultrasound:

  A-scan:
  - Produces a one-dimensional display that represents the major structures of the eye.
  - Now almost exclusively used prior to cataract surgery, to measure the axial length of an eye so that the intraocular lens power can be calculated.

  B-scan:
  - Produces a two-dimensional display allowing localisation and configuration of intraocular structures.
  - Extremely useful when intraocular structures cannot be visualised, e.g. corneal scarring, dense cataract, or vitreous haemorrhage.
  - Intraocular tumours, retinal detachments, and vitreous detachments can be identified by ultrasound, as well as IOFBs, scleritis, and gross pathology at the macula.
  - Although most often used for intraocular diagnosis, it can sometimes be useful in identifying pathology in the extraocular muscles, anterior optic nerve, and sometimes in the orbit.

Lumps on the eye

Typical presentation

There are many different types of "lumps" that can occur on the surface of the eye. However by far the most common are pingueculae and pterygia. Both occur near the corneal limbus either nasally or temporally (i.e. at around 3 o'clock or 9 o'clock if the cornea is thought of as a clock-face). Both are areas of conjunctival degeneration, probably caused by sunlight (Figure 3.19).

Pingueculum

This is a small rounded area of yellowy tissue adjacent to the cornea. The lumps are of no importance and do not usually

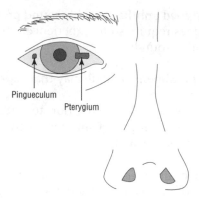

Figure 3.19 Pterygium and pingueculum.

become inflamed. Occasionally patients ask for them to be removed for cosmetic purposes.

Pterygium

This is a small wing of conjunctiva that extends onto the cornea. Rarely this extension can affect the central part of the cornea (i.e. the visual axis). If the pterygium appears to be extending, the patient should be referred. More commonly, they become inflamed and need a short course of topical steroids, i.e. they need referral to an eye casualty department.

Papilloedema

Typical presentation

Papilloedema is defined as optic disc swelling caused by raised intracranial pressure. The other causes of disc swelling which are not due to raised intracranial pressure should **not** be called papilloedema. Papilloedema itself does not cause visual loss although occasionally patients describe momentary visual obscurations. Symptoms tend to occur because of the raised intracranial pressure, e.g. headache or nausea, rather than from the papilloedema itself. However if papilloedema is prolonged the optic discs will become atrophic and visual acuity will decline.

Principles of treatment

1 As mentioned above papilloedema is optic disc swelling due to raised intracranial pressure and therefore it is important to try to rule out other causes of optic disc swelling.
2 If the patient truly has raised intracranial pressure they need immediate referral to a neurologist, not an ophthalmologist.

How and what to do

1 Papilloedema is usually asymptomatic and unlikely to be diagnosed on the history. However the possibility of raised intracranial pressure may well come from the history, e.g. headache worse in the mornings, headache worse when straining, nausea, and vomiting.
2 If the patient's history is suggestive of raised intracranial pressure then a full history and examination will be needed to elucidate any underlying cause.
3 If the visual acuity is found to be down in one or both eyes and/or there is an RAPD, then other causes of disc swelling should be considered such as:
    – AION (consider an underlying temporal arteritis).
    – Optic neuritis (is there pain on eye movements?).
    – CRVO (are there scattered haemorrhages all over the posterior pole?)
4 Remember to check eye movements as raised intracranial pressure can cause VIth nerve palsies. This results in a unilateral or bilateral reduction in the ability to abduct the eye, i.e. the eye cannot "look out".
5 Check the visual fields by confrontation and/or a small target (such as the end of a hat pin).
6 If there is a possibility of raised intracranial pressure:
    – The pupils should not be dilated pharmacologically.
    – The patient can be examined in a darkened room to try to improve the view.
    – Gross papilloedema is usually obvious, the disc appears to be coming towards you and there is no optic cup. There may be scattered haemorrhages around the disc — they should be close to the disc.
    – More subtle disc swelling is much harder to detect as many

normal discs appear to have blurred disc margins (usually long-sighted people).
- Look for venous pulsation of the central retinal vein. The vein is the larger of the two vessels at the disc and it is slightly darker than the artery. **If venous pulsations are present papilloedema is very unlikely.**
- It is important not to make the diagnosis of papilloedema on this sign alone as around 30% of normals have no spontaneous venous pulsations.
- An important feature of papilloedema is that **both** optic discs are swollen. This is possible, but rare in other causes of optic disc swelling.

7 If papilloedema (or symptoms suggestive of raised intracranial pressure) are present refer urgently to a neurologist.

8 Remember to check the blood pressure to rule out malignant hypertension.

Postoperative problems

Typical presentation

Eye surgery can be thought of in two broad categories: (1) external to the globe, i.e. extraocular, and (2) within the globe, i.e. intraocular. The postoperative problems of these two categories are usually quite different.

Patients can present with decreased vision, increased pain, discharge, increasing redness, suture protrusion or simply because they have forgotten their postoperative instructions.

Principles of treatment

1 Post intraocular surgery problems need to be treated with great care. Any decrease in vision or increase in pain may indicate the presence of intraocular infection (endophthalmitis) — a condition which can wipe out the eye in 24 hours unless treated adequately.

2 Extraocular problems are usually less likely to be sight threatening, however if there is obvious postoperative infection an ophthalmic opinion is necessary.

How and what to do

Extraocular surgery

The problems associated with extraocular surgery tend to follow the principles of any sort of surgery:

- infection
- poor wound healing
- suture problems
- haemorrhage.

1 **Lid surgery:**
   – If a lid wound is infected:
   a Take a swab for culture and sensitivity.
   b Start oral antibiotics, e.g. flucloxacillin 500 mg qds and/or amoxicillin 500 mg tds for 1 week. If the patient is penicillin sensitive use erythromycin 500 mg qds for 1 week.
   c Antibiotic ointment or drops are not of great value in these circumstances.
   d With any lid infection it is important to determine if the patient is developing a preseptal or orbital cellulitis. The signs and symptoms of these are discussed on pages 93–96, but refer to an ophthalmologist if the vision is affected, the patient is systemically unwell or pyrexial, or if the patient is a child. The patient with a lid wound infection needs daily review until symptoms and signs improve.
   – Poor wound healing may be because of poor wound construction, infection, or rubbing by the patient. If the wound is gaping or looks unsightly, discuss with the ophthalmologist in charge of the patient.
   – Suture problems are not uncommon. Most lid sutures are removed at 2 weeks. If a suture is causing irritation by rubbing onto the eye it can be shortened.
2 **Lacrimal surgery:**
   – These patients may have a skin wound after surgery and any problems are dealt with in a similar manner to those described for lid surgery.
   – Part or all of the operation is performed via the nose and there is the possibility of secondary nasal haemorrhage.
   – If a patient presents with nasal bleeding after having had lacrimal surgery ask how much and for how long, check their pulse, and BP. The haemorrhage should be treated

like any nose bleed, i.e. pinching the nose, head backwards and packing if necessary.
- If the bleeding cannot be stopped refer to an ENT surgeon immediately.
- Once the haemorrhage has been stopped refer to an ophthalmologist, as the usual cause of a secondary haemorrhage is infection.

3 **Squint surgery:**
- Although planned as an extraocular procedure, it is not uncommon for microperforation of the globe during muscle reattachment. Therefore if a postoperative squint patient complains of decreased vision, redness and pain (i.e. possible endophthalmitis), or increased floaters and a curtain coming over their vision (i.e. possible retinal detachment), refer at once.
- Minor problems after squint surgery include redness, discomfort, and protruding sutures. As long as these are not too troublesome they can be left to the next eye outpatients department appointment.
- Very occasionally a muscle can slip back or off the area onto which it was sutured, which may cause an obvious cosmetic problem or double vision in one particular direction. These need immediate referral as urgent operative exploration is needed.

Intraocular surgery

As endophthalmitis is such a devastating complication, any patient with a red, sore or sticky eye who has had recent intraocular surgery needs to be seen by an ophthalmologist as soon as possible. Most of these will not be endophthalmitis, but in the occasional one that is, early diagnosis and treatment may be sight saving.

1 **Cataract surgery:**
In general, postoperative cataract patients should not experience pain. If they do complain of pain (rather then mild irritation) they should be referred to an ophthalmologist immediately. The commonest serious complications are:
- Postoperative endophthalmitis. This presents with rapidly decreasing vision, increasing pain, and redness — anyone with these symptoms needs immediate ophthalmic referral. More advanced signs include a reactive pupillary defect, corneal clouding, and loss of the red reflex. There may be a hypopyon (a collection of neutrophils that accumulate in the base of the anterior chamber like a snowdrift).

- Postoperative uveitis. There is a normal inflammatory response after surgery (i.e. a mild uveitis) which is why topical steroids are given postoperatively. If this uveitis is more severe the patient will complain of decreasing vision, increasing pain, and redness. The signs and symptoms of severe (but sterile) uveitis are the same as those of endophthalmitis and so urgent ophthalmic opinion is again mandatory.
- The most important late complication (i.e. from around 6 weeks onward) is retinal detachment. This presents as an increase in floaters followed by a "curtain" coming over the vision. Patients need same-day referral.

2 Trabeculectomy:
- This involves creating a fistula between the anterior chamber and the subconjunctival space in an attempt to reduce the IOP.
- In the short term, endophthalmitis and uveitis are possible and should be referred with the same urgency.
- Because a fistula is being formed the risk of intraocular infection remains long after the initial surgery (unlike with cataract surgery where the wound is healed in about 6 weeks). Any patient with a red or sticky eye (even without any signs of intraocular infection) and who has had a trabeculectomy needs same-day ophthalmic referral.

3 Retinal detachment surgery:
- Again both endophthalmitis and uveitis can occur following RD surgery and need immediate referral.
- To re-attach the retina an intraocular gas is sometimes injected into the eye. This gas usually lasts between 2 and 4 weeks and gradually dissipates. In the acute phase it can cause the IOP to rise, the eye will become very painful and the vision decline — the patient may vomit. This requires immediate referral. Patients should be told not to fly when they have an intraocular gas bubble as the change in pressure can cause it to expand and increase the IOP suddenly.
- Occasionally the gas lasts longer than 4 weeks and the patient is troubled by a persistent bubble in their vision. All the patient needs is reassurance that the bubble will disappear soon.
- Often during RD surgery, a buckle is attached to the eye. A buckle is an explant stitched to the sclera to help re-attach the retina. Occasionally, the buckle itself can cause inflammation, become infected, or extrude through the conjunctiva. If any of these problems arise then contact your local eye unit for advice.

– Long-term problems of RD surgery include re-detachment —
  most patients are aware of the symptoms of this and attend
  their eye department automatically — and the development
  of cataract.

Subconjunctival haemorrhage (SCH)

Typical presentation

This occurs when a small blood vessel ruptures beneath the
conjunctiva and it can spread quite easily within this plane.
Patients complain of a rapid onset of a red patch covering the
white areas of the eye, which can vary in size from pinpoint to
the complete subconjunctival space.

Principles of treatment

1 Reassure.
2 Rule out an underlying cause.

How and what to do

1 Subconjunctival haemorrhage is often quite alarming in its
  appearance and rapidity of onset. The patient often needs
  reassurance that nothing serious is wrong with their eye.
2 Check for raised blood pressure — this is one of the few significant correlations with SCH.
3 If the patient is on warfarin check the INR.
4 Explain to the patient that it is really like a very prominent bruise,
  i.e. it will turn yellowy in colour in a few days and will be gone
  after a week.

Section 4
What's left

Optics and refraction for beginners

Although a good knowledge of optics and refraction is essential for ophthalmologists and optometrists, it is unusual for practitioners outside these spheres to need more than a basic knowledge. It is useful to anyone dealing with patients with eye disease to be able to have a simple understanding of the characteristics of the different refractive states and what diseases are associated with them.

The term "refraction" may be confusing, as in scientific terms it means the change in direction of light as it passes from one medium to another. What is a little confusing is that, in clinical practice, "having a refraction" is also used to mean both the act of having a sight test and the result of that sight test, i.e. the overall strength and direction of the individual's refractive error. The glasses that someone needs to correct their refractive error is called their prescription.

1 **Emmetropia:**
   - If an individual has no refractive error, they are called **emmetropic**. The notation for this is a zero, i.e. "0".
2 **Myopia:**
   - If an individual is **shortsighted** this means that an image is focused in front of their retina (it can be thought of as a situation where the eye is too long).
   - This means that they need to wear lenses that allow the focus to be pushed back and onto the retina — this requires **concave** lenses.
   - The conventional notation for concave lenses is a negative sign, i.e. "−" and those who need −ve lenses to correct their refractive error are called **myopes**. The more negative the number the more shortsighted the wearer is.
   - Myopes read better if they bring things closer to their eyes (hence the name shortsighted). They sometimes find it more comfortable to read when they take their distance glasses off.
   - Myopic glasses make the wearer's eyes look smaller. If they are removed, objects viewed through them will look **smaller.**
   - Myopes are at higher risk of retinal detachments (the more myopic, the higher the risk), possibly of primary open angle glaucoma and of early onset macular degeneration.
3 **Hypermetropia:**
   - If an individual is **longsighted** then an image is focused behind the retina (the eye is too short).

- Corrective lenses are needed to bring the image forward onto the retina — this requires **convex** lenses.
- The notation for convex lenses is a plus sign, i.e. "+", and those that require plus lenses are **hypermetropes**. The higher the plus the greater the hypermetropia.
- Low hypermetropes can partially overcome their refractive error by making their natural lens thicker (called **accommodation**) but they need reading glasses at a much younger age than emmetropes.
- Hypermetropic spectacles magnify the wearer's eyes. If they are removed, objects viewed through them will look **bigger**.
- High hypermetropes have small crowded eyes and are therefore at more risk of closed angle glaucoma. Hypermetropia can be a problem in children and is an important factor in some types of convergent squint.

4 Astigmatism:
- The eye is not a perfect sphere (it is often described as rugby ball shaped rather than football shaped). Astigmatism is a measurement of how much the eye deviates from being a perfect sphere — if it was a perfect sphere the astigmatism would be zero.
- Most people have both their main refractive error, i.e. myopia or hypermetropia (known as the spherical error), and astigmatism on top of this.
- The astigmatic error is measured in a similar fashion to the spherical, i.e. the larger the number the greater the lens power needed to correct it.
- If the astigmatic error focuses an image in front of the retina it is called myopic astigmatism, if behind the retina it is hypermetropic astigmatism. But of course astigmatism occurs only in a single direction and this direction is known as the axis of the astigmatism.
- Thus astigmatism is defined in terms of its sign (−ve or +ve), its strength (0.5, 1.0, 1.75, etc) and its direction (90°, 65°, etc.).

5 Accommodation:
- This is the ability of the natural lens to change shape and allow the image of a close object to be focused onto the retina. Thus to be able to read we need to use the accommodative properties of the lens.
- As we get older this accommodation power of the lens is gradually lost and this is called **presbyopia**.

- Emmetropes tend to have the first symptoms of presbyopia at around the age of 45. They compensate for it by holding print farther away from their eyes. Eventually the print cannot be held far enough away and they consult their optometrist who will prescribe simple "+" lenses to give the extra focusing power (these are what are known as "reading glasses"). At around 55 years of age the accommodation of the natural lens is almost completely gone and reading glasses will not need further change (this usually settles at around +3).
- Myopes and hypermetropes go through the same process but because of the different optical properties of their eyes presbyopia has different effects. Generally myopes need reading glasses at an older age than emmetropes while hypermetropes need reading glasses at a younger age.
- In some patients early cataract causes lens thickening rather than lens opacity and this can allow the patient to discard their reading glasses and read without any correction. This is usually temporary: as the cataract progresses it becomes increasingly opacified.
6 **Correction of refractive error:**
- Refractive error can be corrected with glasses or contact lenses — contact lenses are not used for presbyopia as it would blur the patient's distance vision.
- Increasingly refractive errors are being (usually permanently) corrected by laser treatment of the cornea. Until recently this was only available for myopia but it is now used for hypermetropia and astigmatism. It is important to remember that correction of myopic refractive error will hasten the need for reading glasses.
- Cataract surgery can leave the eye in a number of refractive states:
  a Pseudophakic means the eye has an intraocular lens.
  b Aphakia means there is no lens natural or artificial.
  c Astigmatism can be induced by cataract surgery, secondary to the incision made to remove the cataract. This is now less of a problem because of small incision surgery.

Guidelines for blind and partial sight registration

The guidelines for registering someone as blind or partially sighted are defined by The National Assistance Act 1948. A patient can be certified blind if they are "so blind that they cannot do any work for which eyesight is essential". Therefore, the main consideration is visual acuity. Work relates to any work and not the patient's current occupation. Any other physical or mental difficulties should not be considered in the decision.

Visual acuity is defined as the best corrected visual acuity monocularly or binocularly. That is to say if a patient has lost sight in one eye but the fellow eye has good vision then the patient is **not** eligible to be registered partially sighted or blind.

An individual can only be registered blind or partially sighted by a consultant ophthalmologist and may need referral for this (although it is of course voluntary). This registration is made on form BD8.

Who should be certified blind

Patients who are registered as blind fall into three categories:

1 Patients whose vision is less than 3/60 on the Snellen chart in both eyes.
2 Patients whose vision is less than 6/60 but better than 3/60 if they also have significant field loss, e.g. glaucoma.
3 Patients whose vision is better than 6/60 but who have significant field loss, especially inferior field loss, e.g. glaucoma patients, diabetic patients after photocoagulation.

Who should be certified partially sighted

There is no legal definition for partially sighted. The guidelines suggest that a patient is partially sighted if they are "substantially and permanently handicapped by defective vision caused by congenital defect, illness or injury".

The following guidelines are used to register someone as partially sighted:

1 Patients whose vision is less than 6/60 but better than 3/60 with full field in both eyes.
2 Patients whose vision is up to 6/24 with moderate contraction of field, have media opacities, or are aphakic in both eyes.
3 Patients whose vision is up to 6/18 if there is a gross loss of field, e.g. heminopia, glaucoma, retinitis pigmentosa in both eyes.

Infants and children

1 Infants less than 4 years of age with congenital or acquired visual field loss should be registered as partially sighted.
2 Infants over 4 years of age should be registered according to Snellen acuity as defined above.

People who are certified as partially sighted are entitled to most of the same benefits as those who are certified as blind. All those who are registered should receive a visit from the social worker in their area or hospital. The concessions and benefits available depend on the patient's other circumstances and it is important that the patient makes contact with the social worker so that the appropriate benefits for the patient can be assessed.

If patient needs to find out more they can contact "The Benefit Enquiry Line" on 0800 882200 or patients with speech or hearing problems can use a text phone and dial 0800 243355. Alternatively, the Royal National Institute for the Blind (RNIB) can be contacted (see page 205).

Vision and driving

After having an eye condition diagnosed, many patients can be confused and worried regarding their eligibility to drive. Losing a driving licence can seriously affect livelihood, independence, and enjoyment of life. However, a driver with poor eyesight is a potential danger to other road users and a firm but sympathetic approach needs to be taken.

A simple rule for patients or practitioners is that if there is a query regarding visual requirements to drive the DVLA must be consulted. It is they, rather than ophthalmologists, who make the decision. The DVLA should always be informed when a potentially sight-threatening condition is newly diagnosed, even if the disease appears to have no effect on the vision. Similarly they should also be informed if there is a change in a pre-existing condition.

The legal visual requirements for driving are:

1 The ability to read a standard number plate in good daylight from 20.5 m (67 feet) with best correction.
2 Visual acuity of 6/12 in the better eye (i.e. only having one eye is not in itself a barrier to driving).

3 A field of vision between 120° on the horizontal and 20° above and below the horizontal from fixation.

In practice most people are tested using the number plate at 20.5 m and it is only if there is the possibility of a visual problem (e.g. macular degeneration or glaucoma) that the latter two are tested, usually by an ophthalmologist.

It is the responsibility of patients to inform the DVLA about any visual defects. The practitioner should strongly advise them to do so. If this is a problem, the GMC have produced guidelines for this. Before they notify the DVLA patients should have a refraction and field test with their optometrist. If the vision cannot be corrected with glasses or there is field defect the patient should be referred to an ophthalmologist for further management. Until then the patient should be advised not to drive. The DVLA will contact the ophthalmologist for a report on the patient.

The legal requirements for driving heavy goods vehicles and passenger service vehicles are strict, although to some extent they depend on the size of the vehicle. The basic requirements are:

1 At least 6/9 Snellen visual acuity in the better eye and at least 6/12 in the other eye with best correction.
2 No worse than 3/60 in each eye without glasses or contact lenses.
3 A full visual field between 120° on the horizontal and 20° from fixation.

If you or the patient are unsure or require further help, the DVLA medical advisory department can be contacted on 01792 783693.

Useful addresses and web sites for patients

General contacts

Two useful starting places for self-help groups in the UK are *www.patient.co.uk* and *www.omni.co.uk*

Action for Blind People   14–16 Verney Road
London
SE16 3DZ
http://www.demon.co.uk/afbp

Blindcare	Springhill
	Kennylands Road
	Sonning Common
	Reading
	RG4 9JT
	www.btinternet.com/~blindcare/
British Telecom Age	9th Floor, Burne House
and Disability Unit	Bell Street
	London
	NW1 5BZ
British Wireless for	Gabriel House
the Blind	34 New Road
	Chatham
	Kent
	ME4 4QR
Deafblind UK	100 Bridge Street
	Peterborough
	PE1 1DY
Fight For Sight	Institute of Ophthalmology
	Bath St
	London
	EC1V 9EL
Guide Dogs for the	Hillfields
Blind Association	Burfield Common
	Reading
	RG7 3YG
	http://www.gdba.org.uk
Moorfields Eye Hospital	City Road
	London
	EC1V 2PD
	www.moorfields.com
National Federation for	Unity House
the Blind in the UK	Smyth Street
	Wakefield
	West Yorkshire
	WF1 1ER

The Partially Sighted Society	9 Plato Place 72–74 St Dionis Road London SW6 4TU
Royal National Institute for the Blind	224 Great Portland Street London W1N 6AA http://www.rnib.org.uk
Royal National College for the Blind	College Road Hereford HR1 1EB http://www.rncb.ac.uk
Scottish National Federation for the Welfare of the Blind	50 Gillespie Crescent Edinburgh EH10 4HZ
Talking Newspaper Enterprises Limited	National Recording Centre Heathfield Sussex TN21 8DB http://www.tnauk.org.uk

Specific disease groups

Allergy

British Allergy Foundation
Deepdene House
30 Bellegrove Road
Welling
Kent
DA16 3PY

Ankylosing spondylitis

National Ankylosing Spondylitis
Society
PO Box 179
Mayfield
East Sussex
TN20 6ZL

Diabetes	British Diabetic Association 10 Queen Anne Street London W1M 0BD www.diabetes.org.uk
Bullous pemphigoid	Bullous Pemphigoid Support Group 17 Barley Mount Redhills Exeter EX14 1RP
Herpetic disease	The Herpes Virus Association and Shingles Support Society 41 North Road London N7 9DP
HIV disease	Terence Higgins Trust 52–54 Grays Inn Road London WC1X 8JU
Glaucoma	International Glaucoma Association c/o King's College Hospital Denmark Hill London SE5 9RS
Marfan's syndrome	Marfan Association Rochester House 5 Aldershot Road Fleet Hants GU13 9NG
Multiple sclerosis	Multiple Sclerosis Society 25 Effie Road Fulham London SW16 1EE

Myasthenia gravis	Myasthenia Gravis Association Keynes House Chester Park Alfreton Road Derby DE21 4AS
Neurofibromatosis	Neurofibromatosis Association 82 London Road Kingston on Thames Surrey KT2 6PX http://www.users.zetnet.co.uk. neurofibromatosis
Pituitary disease	The Pituitary Foundation 17/18 The Courtyard Woodlands, Bradley Stoke Bristol BS32 4NQ
Postherpetic neuralgia	Pain Society 9 Bedford Square London WC1B 3RA
Progressive supranuclear palsy	PSP Europe Association The Old Rectory Wappenham Towcester Northants NN12 9SQ
Psoriasis	Psoriasis Association 7 Milton Street Northampton NN2 7JG
Thyroid eye disease	TED Head Office 34 Fore Street Chudleigh Devon TQ13 0HX

Sjögren's syndrome	British Sjögren's Syndrome Association
	Unit 1, Manor Workshops
	Nailsea Wall Lane
	West End
	Nailsea
	Bristol
	BS48 4DD
Systemic lupus	Lupus UK
erythematosus (SLE)	St James's House
	Eastern Road
	Romford
	Essex
	RM1 3NH
Stroke	The Stroke Association
	Stroke House
	Whitecross Street
	London
	EC1Y 8JJ

Eye sites (some useful eye-related web sites for the clinician)

Some of these web sites are disease orientated, providing descriptions and pictures of various eye diseases, some contain details of research and others are really directed at patient information. Almost all have links to other sites — the depth and breadth of eye information on the internet is breathtaking

Access to Medline	www.bmj.com
American Academy of Ophthalmology	www.eyenet.org
Cochrane Eyes and Vision	www.archie.ucl.ac.uk
Moorfields Eye Hospital	www.moorfields.com
National Eye Institute (USA)	www.nei.nih.gov
The Royal College of Ophthalmologists	www.rcophth.ac.uk
Schepens Institute	www.eri.harvard.edu
For ophthalmology books	www.bmjbooks.com
	www.amazon.com
Other useful sites	www.onsu.edu/cliniweb
	www.eyemax.com

Glossary of ophthalmic terms and abbreviations

This section is a description of some of the terms and abbreviations you may come across in ophthalmic notes and letters and which can be impossible to decipher!

AAU	Acute anterior uveitis. This is a sterile inflammation of the anterior eye which may be idiopathic or secondary to a systemic disease.
AC	Anterior chamber.
ACAG	Acute closed angle glaucoma.
Acanthamoeba keratitis	Amoebic infection of the cornea usually occurs in contact lens wearers who have washed their lenses in tap water. Occasionally seen after corneal abrasions caused by agricultural implements.
AION	Anterior ischaemic optic neuropathy.
Amaurosis fugax	Fleeting loss of vision.
Amblyopia	Amblyopia is decreased visual acuity without any detectable organic disease of the eye.
AMD (or ARMD)	Age-related macular degeneration (previously called senile macular degeneration — SMD).
Amsler chart	Grid used to detect distortion caused by macular pathology.
Anisocoria	A difference in size of the two pupils.
APD	Afferent pupillary defect (also called a Marcus Gunn pupil). This term is used but should not be, as afferent papillary defects can only be elicited by shining a light from one eye to the other, i.e. it is a relative afferent pupillary defect (RAPD).
ARMD (or AMD)	Age-related macular degeneration.
BCC	Basal cell carcinoma.
BCL	Bandage contact lens. This is a non-refractive contact lens used to protect the cornea.
BD8	The form that is used to register someone blind or partially sighted.
BEQ	Means "Both Eyes Quiet", i.e. not red and with no anterior chamber activity.
Bell's phenomenon	A normal reflex that involves the eye rolling upwards when the lids are closed.

Blepharitis	Inflammation of the eyelid margins leading to gritty, irritable, red lids and conjunctiva.
Blepharospasm	Forcible closure of the lids.
Blow-out fracture	Fracture of the floor of the orbit.
BRAO	Branch retinal artery occlusion.
BRVO	Branch retinal vein occlusion.
BTX	Botulinum toxin.
Canthus	This is an anatomical description of the lateral and medial extent of the external eye and is where the upper and lower lids meet. Thus there is a medial and lateral canthus.
Cat	Short for cataract.
CFB	Corneal foreign body.
CFS (or CFs)	Counting fingers vision — the patient can distinguish the examiner's fingers held in front of their eye(s).
Chalazion	A lid lump caused by enlargement of a meibomian gland (pleural chalazia).
Chemosis	Conjunctival oedema.
Chlor	Abbreviation for chloramphenicol.
CL	Contact lens. May be hard or soft — the latter are associated with a much higher risk of microbial keratitis as they are worn for much longer periods. Gas permeable lenses are hard but have increased oxygen passage to the cornea.
CLP	Contact lens practitioner — someone who fits and maintains contact lenses.
CMO	Cystoid macular oedema (excess fluid at the macula). The American abbreviation is CME (edema).
CMV	Cytomegalovirus.
COAG	Chronic open angle glaucoma (i.e. POAG).
Coloboma	Notches or fissures of the eye usually congenital in origin.
Cortical blindness	Visual loss due to abnormalities in the visual (occipital) cortex of the brain.
Conj	Abbreviation for conjunctiva.
Conjunctiva	The mucous membrane that covers the anterior globe and lids. Conjunctiva lining the lids is called the tarsal conjunctiva and that lining the globe is the bulbar conjunctiva.
CRAO	Central retinal artery occlusion.
CRVO	Central retinal vein occlusion.
CSR	Central serous retinopathy. This is a condition of unknown aetiology that usually occurs in young males. It is a leakage of fluid under the macula.
CWS	Cotton-wool spots.
Cyclo	Abbreviation for cyclopentolate.
Cycloplegic	A drug that causes ciliary muscle paralysis (and usually dilates the pupil).

Dacrocystitis	Inflammation of the lacrimal sac.
DCR	Dacrocystorhinostomy (an operation that produces a fistula between the lacrimal sac and nasal mucosa, allowing bypass of a nasolacrimal duct obstruction).
Dendritic ulcer	Clinical description of the branching ulcer seen with corneal infection by the herpes simplex virus (herpes simplex keratitis).
Diplopia	Double vision.
DR	Diabetic retinopathy.
ECCE	Extracapsular cataract extraction — removal of the cataract but leaving the natural covering of the lens behind (also known as the capsular bag), to reduce complications.
Ectropion	Turning out of the lid.
ELO	Early lens opacities, i.e. early cataract.
Emmetropia	When an eye has no refractive error.
Endophthalmitis	Inflammation (usually infective) throughout the whole of the inner eye.
Enophthalmos	Recession of the eye into the orbit.
Entropion	Turning in of the lid so that the lashes may abrade the cornea.
EOM	Extraocular **muscles** or extraocular **movements**.
Epiphora	Eye watering secondary to lacrimal drainage abnormalities.
Episcleritis	Inflammation of the tissues overlying the sclera.
ESR	Erythrocyte sedimentation rate.
EUA	Examination under anaesthetic.
Exophthalmos	Proptosis caused by thyroid eye disease.
Exposure keratopathy	Corneal damage caused by an abnormal lid closure.
Extraocular	Outside the eye, e.g. extraocular muscles are the muscles attached to the outside of the globe.
FB	Foreign body.
Floaters	Term used to describe opacities in the vitreous jelly (perceived by the patient to be floating in front of their vision).
FML	Abbreviation sometimes used for g. fluoromethalone.
Fornix	This is where the conjunctiva is reflected back on itself to form a "pocket". This occurs on the underside of the upper lid (the superior fornix) and lower lid (inferior fornix).
Fundoscopy	Examining the ocular fundus, i.e. the retina, optic disc and macula.
Fundus	Generic term to describe the retina, optic disc and macula.
G. or g.	Stands for Guttae and means drops.
GCA	Giant cell arteritis (temporal arteritis).

Globe	The term used to describe the eyeball itself.
GOS 18	The form used by optometrists to refer a patient to a general practitioner.
GPL	Gas permeable lens — a type of hard contact lens.
HA	Abbreviation for homatropine.
Hemianopia	Loss of half of the visual field.
HES	Hospital eye service, i.e. a hospital eye department.
HMS (or HMs)	Hand movement vision — the patient can see the examiner's hand moving in front of their eye(s).
HPM	Abbreviation sometimes used for hypromellose.
HSK	Herpes simplex keratitis. This is corneal infection with the herpes simplex virus and its appearance on the cornea is described as a dendritic ulcer.
Hypermetropia	"Long-sightedness".
Hyphaema	Blood in the anterior chamber of the eye.
Hypopyon	Pus (i.e. inflammatory material) in the anterior chamber of the eye.
HZO	Herpes zoster ophthalmicus. This is shingles affecting the ophthalmic (first) division of the trigeminal nerve.
ICCE	Intracapsular cataract extraction — removal of cataract and its coverings in total.
Injected eye	This simply means that the eye is red.
Intraocular	Inside the eye.
IO	Intraocular.
IOFB	Intraocular foreign body.
IOP	Intraocular pressure.
IR	Inferior rectus muscle.
Ishihara plates	Colour vision testing plates.
KCS	Keratoconjunctivitis sicca (dry eye).
Keratitis	A generic term for corneal inflammation.
KP	Keratic precipitates (inflammatory cells on the corneal endothelium).
Lagophthalmos	Incomplete eyelid closure.
LCS or RCS	Left or right **convergent** squint. Convergent means that the affected eye is looking inward (i.e. towards the nasal side) compared to the other one.
LDS or RDS	Left or right **divergent** squint. Divergent means that the affected eye is looking outward (i.e. towards the temporal side) compared to the other one.
Limbus	The part of the eye where the sclera meets the cornea (and where the conjunctiva inserts).
LR	Lacteral rectus muscle.
LVA	Low visual aids (magnifying glasses, telescopes, etc.).

Meibomian glands	Glands in the eyelids that normally secrete lipid into the tear film.
Metamorphopsia	The perception of distortion of straight lines usually caused by pathology under the macula.
Minims	Single-use eye drop sachets.
Miosis	Small pupil (e.g. in Horner's syndrome or after pilocarpine instillation).
MR	Medial rectus muscle.
Mydriasis	Dilated pupil.
Myokymia	Involuntary twitching of the orbicularis muscle.
Myopia	"Short-sightedness".
NLD	Nasolacrimal duct.
NPL	No perception of light — the patient is unable to detect a bright light held in front of their eyes(s).
NS	Nuclear sclerosis — a type of cataract.
NVM	Neovascular membrane. Usually subretinal (especially around the macula).
Occ.	Ointment.
OD	Right eye.
Ophthalmia neonatorum	Conjunctivitis within the first month of life.
Ophthalmologist	Medical practitioner trained to diagnose and treat eye disorders medically and surgically.
Ophthalmoscopy	Viewing the eye with the ophthalmoscope (direct or indirect).
Optic chiasm	The area where nerve fibres from both eyes cross and pass on to the brain.
Optician	See optometrist.
Optometrist	Practitioners who perform eye tests — usually in commercial practice. This is now the preferred term for ophthalmic opticians. Dispensing opticians are those who make spectacles but do not perform eye tests.
Orthoptist	Practitioners trained to test eye movements and their disorders and to supervise amblyopia detection and treatment — either in a hospital eye department or in a community setting.
OS	Left eye.
PCO	Posterior capsule opacification. This is the term used to describe thickening of the lens capsule after cataract surgery.
PDR	Proliferative diabetic retinopathy.
PDS	Pigment dispersion syndrome (raised IOP caused by blockage of the trabecular meshwork by pigment shed from the iris).
PE	Abbreviation for phenylephrine.
PEE	Punctuate epithelial erosions (corneal).
PERL	Pupils equal (in size) and reactant to light.
PERLA	Pupils equal and reactant to light and accommodation.

PI	Peripheral iridectomy.
PL (or POL)	Perception of light — the patient can see a bright light held in front of their eye(s).
PMR	Polymyalgia rheumatica.
POAG	Primary open angle glaucoma.
Posterior pole	Describes the very posterior part of the eye centred on the macula.
Proptosis	Protrusion of the globe.
PRP	Pan-retinal photocoagulation.
PSCLO	Posterior subcapsular lens opacities — a type of cataract.
Ptosis	Drooping of the upper lid.
PVD	Posterior vitreous detachment.
PVR	Proliferative vitreoretinopathy — this is fibrous tissue forming within the vitreous usually after failed retinal detachment surgery.
PXF	Pseudoexfoliation (sometimes abbreviated to PXE — but this can be confused with pseudoxanthoma elasticum).
RAPD	Reactive afferent papillary defect (also called a Marcus Gunn pupil).
RBN	Retrobulbar neuritis (optic neuritis).
RD	Retinal detachment.
RES	Recurrent epithelial abrasion syndrome.
RP	Retinitis pigmentosa.
RR	Red reflex or sometimes used as an abbreviation for rust ring.
Rubeosis	New blood vessels forming in the drainage angle of the eye, i.e. covering the trabecular meshwork. If the intraocular pressure rises this is called rubeotic glaucoma.
SCC	Squamous cell carcinoma.
SCH	Subconjunctival haemorrhage.
Schirmer's	A test of tear production.
Scleritis	Inflammation of the outer coat of the eye (sclera).
Scotoma	This is a small area of visual field loss.
SMD	Senile macular degeneration — now called age-related macular degeneration.
SO	Superior oblique muscle.
SR	Superior rectus muscle.
SRNVM	Subretinal neovascular membrane.
STFB	Subtarsal foreign body.
Strabismus	Another name for squint.
Subtarsal	Underneath the lid.
Suppression	Ability of the brain to "ignore" one of the images when diplopia occurs. Usually occurs in children.
Synaechia	Abnormal connections between the iris and surrounding tissue, e.g. anterior synaechia is a connection to the cornea, posterior is to the lens. Plural synaechiae.

TA	Temporal arteritis (also called giant cell or cranial arteritis) or sometimes is an abbreviation for the temporal arteries themselves.
TAB	Temporal artery biopsy.
Tarsorraphy	Therapeutic closure of the eyelids to protect the cornea.
TED	Thyroid eye disease.
TFBUT	Tear film break-up time — used to determine how rapidly the tears are evaporating from the cornea.
TIA	Transient ischaemic attack.
Trabeculectomy	An operation that attempts to reduce the IOP in patients with glaucoma by creating an aqueous fistula between the anterior chamber and subconjuntival space.
Trichiasis	Lashes rubbing on the cornea.
Trop	Abbreviation for tropicamide.
Uveitis	Inflammation of the uveal tract (iris, ciliary body, and choroid). May be acute or chronic and often described in relation to the part of the eye it affects, i.e. anterior, intermediate or posterior.
VA	Visual acuity.
Visual cortex	This is the part of the brain that deals with vision. It is situated in the occipital lobes of the brain and therefore also called the occipital cortex.
Vitritis	Visible inflammatory cells and debris within the vitreous jelly.

Reduced Snellen Chart

- to be read at $\sim\frac{1}{3}$ m
- patient to use reading glasses if he/she normally does

Equivalent to

6/60	T	V	O
6/36	X	H	A
6/24	A	X	T
6/18	H	O	U
6/12	x	u	H
6/9	T	o	v
6/9	H	x	u
6/6			
6/6			
6/4			
6/4			

Index

Page numbers in *italics* refer to tables or boxed material, and those in **bold**, to figures